INTENSIVE CARE

Medical Ethics
and the
Medical Profession

Robert Zussman

The University of Chicago Press
Chicago and London

INTENSIVE CARE

The University of Chicago Press, Chicago 60637
The University of Chicago Press, Ltd., London
© 1992 by The University of Chicago
All rights reserved. Published 1992
Paperback edition 1994
Printed in the United States of America

00 99 98 97 96   5 4 3 2

ISBN 0–226–99634–4 (cloth)
ISBN 0–226–99635–2 (paper)

Library of Congress Cataloging-in-Publication Data

Zussman, Robert.
    Intensive care : medical ethics and the medical profession /
Robert Zussman.
        p.   cm.
    Includes index.
    1. Critical care medicine—Moral and ethical aspects.   I. Title.
    [DNLM: 1. Critical Care.   2. Ethics, Medical.   W 50 Z96i]
RC86.95.Z87   1992
174′.24—dc20
DNLM/DLC
for Library of Congress   91–36919
                                                                              CIP

⊗ The paper used in this publication meets the minimum requirements of the
American National Standard for Information Sciences—Permanence of Paper
for Printed Library Materials, ANSI Z39.48–1984.

Contents

Acknowledgments

Intensive Care reports the results of extensive field research in two hospitals. Although I often found the research fascinating, I would not say that I exactly enjoyed it. In hospitals, particularly in intensive care units, sickness and death are constant presences. As in much fieldwork, I often found that long hours yielded only the slimmest of insights. Not least—and like field-workers more generally—I found myself in the uncomfortable position of being an intruder, pestering already tired doctors and nurses with what must have seemed endless questions, imposing on patients and their families during the most trying of circumstances. I marveled then and I marvel now that they treated me with considerable courtesy and generosity. And I regret that I have nothing to offer in return except my gratitude. At very least, my first thanks must go to those doctors, nurses, patients, and families whom the canons of confidentiality prevent me from naming but without whom I could not have completed this project.

Sherry Brandt-Rauf, Stephanie Kiceluk, Connie Park, David Rothman, and Sheila Rothman, all of the Center for the Study of Society and Medicine at Columbia University, lent wisdom and encouragement at the beginning of the project. Dan Clawson, Mary Ann Clawson, Eliot Freidson, John Gagnon, Herb Gans, David Halle, David Rothman, Michael Schwartz, Judy Tanur, Dan Teres, Nancy Tomes, and Eviatar Zerubavel read and commented on all or part of the manuscript as did two remarkably thorough anonymous reviewers for the University of Chicago Press and two cohorts of excellent Stony Brook graduate students in my seminars on the professions and on field methods. Jonathan Sharpe (who conducted some of the interviews reported in chapter 7), Cathy Marrone, and Sam Lewis provided valuable research assistance. At the University of Chicago Press, Doug Mitchell, Craig Gill, and Jennie Lightner handled the publication process with care and patience. Grants from the National Center for Health Services Re-

search (HS 05548) and the Arthur Vining Davis Foundation made the research both much easier and much better than it would otherwise have been.

Mark Zussman, among other things, edited the entire manuscript. Bernis
Zussman, among other things, asked enough questions but not too many.
Naomi Gerstel, among other things, read many drafts of each chapter, made
me think out the research better, made me think out my arguments better,
kept me from overestimating the significance of what I was finding, kept me
from underestimating the significance of what I was finding, and put up with
me through the whole process.

I began my research soon after the death of my father. I finished writing
soon after the birth of my daughter, Kate. In the midst of a project marked
by a frequent preoccupation with death, there has been both solace and joy
in their reminder that, while the cycles of life do sometimes begin with end-
ings, they may also end with beginnings.

1

Medical Ethics and the Medical Profession

This book is about medical ethics. More specifically, it is about informed consent, the limitation of potentially life prolonging treatment, and the allocation of scarce resources in two intensive care units I studied between 1985 and 1989. This book is about medical ethics, but it is not itself a work of medical ethics. Medical ethics, according to one of its leading practitioners, is a "type of *applied ethics*—the application of general ethical theories, principles, and rules to problems of therapeutic practice, health care delivery, and medical and biological research." [1] Medical ethics is primarily normative. This book is not. Medical ethics addresses matters of right and wrong: how much and what kind of information a patient should receive before going to surgery or before a therapeutic procedure; when it is morally permissible (and when not) to turn off a respirator; who deserves dialysis or the last bed in an intensive care unit when there are fewer dialysis machines or beds available there are patients who need them. Of such matters, this book has little or nothing to add to what others have already said. Rather, this book is about the ways in which right and wrong are interpreted and used—about the ways in which conceptions of right and wrong emerge out of the social situations of patients and their families, of doctors and nurses, from the workings of hospitals and the courts, and then reflect back on those situations. This book is, then, insistently and self-consciously empirical.

I have no quarrel with the questions medical ethicists have asked or, for that matter, with many of the answers they have supplied. Much of the literature of medical ethics is of the very highest quality. The dominant perspectives of medical ethicists are ones that I, for the most part, sympathize with. But we should not imagine that the questions that preoccupy medical ethicists are the only ones we might ask, for in concentrating on questions of how medical decisions should be made, medical ethicists have paid surpris-

---

1. Tom Beauchamp and James F. Childress, *Principles of Biomedical Ethics* (New York: Oxford University Press, 1979), pp. vi–vii.

ingly little attention to how they are in fact made. As a result, medical ethics, and consequently the public policies that medical ethics have helped to shape, have been characterized by striking omissions.

First, medical ethics has fairly consistently ignored the social context in which medical decisions are made. As Renee Fox has observed, medical ethicists have most often conceptualized medical decisions as if they were contracts—rational and voluntary agreements, usually between doctor and patient, acting as independent individuals.[2] They have, for example, stressed the importance of formal procedures in obtaining patients' consent for medical procedures. But at the same time they have ignored both the social forces that shape patients' values and the very real imbalance of influence between patients and their doctors, the very (nonrational) matters that account for patients' willingness to give consent. Medical ethics, in short, has failed to acknowledge that everything in the contract is not contractual.

Second, medical ethics is curiously lacking in self-reflection. Ethics has become a prominent part of the medical landscape—debated in the courts of law and public opinion, taught in medical schools, and applied in hospital wards and physicians' private offices. Medical ethics has its own history. It emerges out of a distinctive set of values and concerns. Yet, with very few exceptions, one will search in vain for any analysis of how medical ethics works in practice.[3] This is a curious omission. It is one thing to enunciate a set of principles, teach them, even see them elaborated into laws and regulations. It is quite another to see how they are honored in hospitals, clinics, and doctors' offices. Medicine, in particular, has a long history of turning to its own purposes the attempts of others to regulate it. Whether it has suc-

2. Renee Fox, *The Sociology of Medicine* (Englewood Cliffs, NJ: Prentice Hall, 1989), p. 229. See also Renee Fox and Judith Swazey, "Medical Morality Is Not Bioethics—Medical Ethics in China and the United States," *Perspectives in Biology and Medicine* 27 (1984): 336–60.

3. For a criticism of medical ethics along similar lines, by a leader from within the field itself, see Leon Kass, "Practicing Ethics: Where's the Action?" *Hastings Center Report*, January/February 1990, pp. 5–12. I should also note that there is a large body of what might be called "descriptive ethics" concentrated particularly in the medical journals. Indeed, I have been much influenced by this literature and rely heavily on it in the pages that follow for discussions of such matters as the frequency with which Do Not Resuscitate orders are issued and the conditions under which physicians seek informed consent. I have, however, also found the literature of descriptive ethics limited in at least two respects. In the first instance, it has been tentative and cautious in making explicit its implications for normative questions with the result that it has exercised only intermittent influence on the more prescriptive brand of medical ethics. In the second instance, the literature has only rarely moved beyond description of ethically relevant practices to an explanation of those practices rooted firmly in an analysis of professional or hospital organization.

ceeded in doing so with the initiatives of medical ethics, we do not know.[4] In short, what is called for is not only a philosophy of medical ethics but a sociology.

Sociology cannot, of course, answer the questions of medical ethics as they have conventionally been posed. Sociology, as Max Weber noted long ago, cannot tell us "whether life is worth living and when."[5] Sociology cannot tell us when we should terminate a medical treatment and when we should continue it. Sociology cannot tell us who should or should not receive dialysis or a heart transplant or even how we should decide such truly weighty matters. The claims of sociology are more modest. But sociology can tell us something.

If sociology cannot tell us how matters of medical ethics should be resolved, it can tell us how, in fact, they are resolved. It can tell us when medical treatments are likely to be terminated or continued, under what conditions, and for what reasons. It can tell us who does receive dialysis or a heart transplant, under what circumstances, by what decision-making process. Perhaps most important, sociology can tell us what values underlie those decisions, how those values articulate with other values, how they emerge from the interests and influence of different groups or organizations, and what in the organization of medicine or American society more generally frustrates the realization of other values. This is not, to be sure, the same as asking whether a life is worth living and when, but they are important issues nonetheless.

If sociology can tell us a good deal about medical ethics, medical ethics can also tell us a good deal about medicine more generally. Insofar as most medical ethicists speculate at all about the origins of their own field, they assume that it is a more or less natural response to the genuinely remarkable development of new medical technologies over the past several decades. And undoubtedly there is some truth in ascribing the recent burst of interest in

4. The work of Lidz, Meisel, and their colleagues stands out as one of the few efforts to answer such questions. See Charles Lidz, Alan Meisel, Marian Osterweis, Janice L. Holden, John H. Marx, and Mark Munetz, "Barriers to Informed Consent," *Annals of Internal Medicine* 1983 (99): 539–43; Charles W. Lidz and Alan Meisel with Janice L. Holden, John H. Marx, and Mark Munetz, "Informed Consent and the Structure of Medical Care," in President's Commission for the Study of Ethical Problems in Medicine and Biomedical and Behavioral Research, *Making Health Care Decisions*, vol. 2: *Appendices, Empirical Studies of Informed Consent* (Washington, DC: Government Printing Office, 1982), pp. 317–410; and Charles Lidz, Alan Meisel, Eviatar Zerubavel, Mary Carter, Regina Sestak, and Loren Roth, *Informed Consent* (New York: Guilford Press, 1984).

5. H. H. Gerth and C. Wright Mills, eds., *From Max Weber* (New York: Oxford University Press, 1946), p. 144.

medical ethics to the development of such technical wonders as artificial hearts, artificial kidneys, and breathing machines. But such an explanation is far too simple. The issues that make up the core of medical ethics as it is conventionally defined—issues around genetic screening, biomedical research, and abortion as well as informed consent, termination of treatment, and the allocation of resources—are nothing less than an arena in which fundamental and competing visions of medicine's future contend. Sociologists of medicine have long been preoccupied with the ability of physicians both to escape a great deal of outside regulation and to impose their own visions of health and illness on a general public. Medical ethics—to state the matter bluntly—is the site at which this long-standing authority of medicine is now being challenged.

The starting point, then, for any sociology of medical ethics must be a recognition that the very field itself is both symptom and, to some degree, cause of the waning of medicine's authority. It was not always thus. At the middle of the nineteenth century, medicine embarked on a century-long march that took it from an only sometimes respectable trade to the very pinnacle of successful professionalism.[6] In the course of this transformation, medicine won not only prestige and income but also the right to determine what was to be considered a medical problem and what not. This is a story often told and need be repeated here only briefly.

At its core, medicine's "professional project" was based on an invocation of science that helped it both to win a monopoly over the market for its services and to convince the American public that those services were essential to good health. So-called regular physicians won the enactment of licensing laws which coupled the right to practice with passage through a certified medical education—thus eliminating the competition of the various self-proclaimed healers, ranging from midwives to often untrained medical sectarians, who had provided an alternative to regular physicians throughout the nineteenth century. At the same time, physicians were able to create a demand for their services by incorporating an ever-expanding roster of human experience and problems—ranging from childbirth to public sanitation—into the realm of medical practice. Often this meant defining as a technical problem what had been or could be defined as a moral problem.

---

6. Four of the most important accounts of medicine's success can be found in Eliot Freidson, *Profession of Medicine* (New York: Harper & Row, 1970); Magali Sarfatti-Larson, *The Rise of Professionalism* (Berkeley: University of California Press, 1977); Peter Conrad and Joseph Schneider, *Deviance and Medicalization* (St. Louis: C. V. Mosby, 1980); and Paul Starr, *The Social Transformation of American Medicine* (New York: Basic Books, 1982).

Consider, for example, abortion—a particularly ironic case in light of the moral fervor that now surrounds it. Throughout most of the nineteenth century abortion was legal, at least until "quickening," the first indication of fetal movement. Moreover, most abortions were probably performed with home remedies and without the supervision of a physician. However, by the end of the nineteenth century medicine had secured the passage of laws making abortion illegal, except in cases where it was deemed medically indicated for the life or health of the mother. As Kristen Luker has observed, physicians successfully "transformed the terms of debate," winning control over the right to abortion by posing the questions surrounding it as ones of medical fact rather than value. Although physicians recognized moral issues in abortion, "they framed their own claim to it as a professional and technical one."[7] This is a process precisely the reverse of that represented by the contemporary rise of medical ethics. It is also a strategy available only to a profession in ascendance.

Since at least the 1960s, however, medicine has not been a profession in ascendance. To be sure, physicians continue to enjoy not only considerable prestige and generous incomes (roughly five times the income of the average full-time wage earner) but also legal protection of their monopoly over their right to practice. Yet, at the same time, it is clear that the political and cultural authority of medicine is waning. While the full dimensions of this process are not yet clear, several observations can be made about its sources.

First, medicine has shared in the general decline in trust of all experts that has characterized the last two and a half decades. Although physicians have fared no worse (and usually better) than courts, politicians, and the military, the proportion of Americans expressing "a great deal of trust" in medicine had nonetheless declined from roughly two-thirds in the mid–1960s to just under one-half by the 1980s.[8]

Second, medicine has become a victim of its own success. Having convinced a public that it is essential to health, medicine has become big business. Since the passage of Medicaid and Medicare in 1965, medical care has assumed a significant place in the federal budget, now accounting for over 11 percent of total expenditures.[9] In private industry, according to one telling calculation, nearly one-tenth of the cost of every car manufactured by the

7. Kristen Luker, *Abortion and the Politics of Motherhood* (Berkeley: University of California Press, 1984), p. 43.

8. *General Social Survey* (Chicago: National Opinion Research Center, 1990).

9. U.S. Bureau of the Census, *Statistical Abstracts of the United States*, 110th ed. (Washington, DC: Government Printing Office, 1990).

Chrysler Corporation in 1982 went to providing health care for the men and women who manufactured it.[10] If, in the 1960s, public policy discussions of medicine were framed in response to questions of improving access to physicians and hospitals, today they are framed around questions of controlling costs. Most important is the introduction of "prospective payments" for hospital costs by Medicare and other third-party payers. Unlike "cost plus" reimbursements, which maximized hospitals' financial incentives to treat patients extensively, prospective payments, which reimburse at a fixed rate determined by the patient's condition on entry to the hospital, attempt to minimize those incentives. Among physicians, the sense of boundless financing for medical care that was characteristic of the late 1960s has given way to a keen sense of the limitations of resources. Unlike the scattered individuals who made up the market for medical services through the first half of the twentieth century, big business and big government are consumers with considerable clout. The escalating costs of medical care have created not only a desire to regulate medicine but also the means to do so.

Third, the slow decline of family physicians and their replacement by the specialist, group practice, and the hospital or clinic have severed many of the personal ties that once bound patients to their doctors. At the same time, whatever the ultimate fate of efforts to control medical costs, Medicare and Medicaid did contribute to patients' sense of entitlement. By removing much of medical care from the realm of charity, they contributed not only to a public perception of rights *to* medical care but also to a demand for rights *in* medical care. This new demand—amounting, according to some, to nothing less than a consumer revolt—includes an insistence on more explanation and greater participation in decision making.[11] Unsatisfied patients have recourse not only to the organizations that employ their physicians but also to third-party payers and to the courts. What was once an intimate relationship has become, increasingly, a bureaucratic one.

This is the context in which medical ethics has emerged. It is a fundamental premise of this book that medical ethics can be understood as an effort to regulate medicine and that this effort is both cause and consequence

10. Jonathon E. Fielding, "Health Promotion and Disease Prevention at the Workplace," in *Annual Review of Public Health* 5 (1984): 237–65.

11. On a consumer revolt in medicine, see Marie R. Haug and Bebe Lavin, *Consumerism in Medicine* (Beverly Hills: Sage, 1983); Leo Reeder, "The Patient as Client-Consumer: Some Observations on the Changing Professional-Client Relationship," *Journal of Health and Social Behavior* (1972) 13: 406–12. For some critical comments on the notion of a consumer revolt, see Eliot Freidson, "The Reorganization of the Medical Profession," *Medical Care Review* (1985) 42: 11–35.

of the waning of medicine's cultural authority.[12] To be sure, medical ethics as an intellectual discipline is at least as old as Hippocrates. But it is only since about 1960 that medical ethics has also become a social movement.

Much of the impetus for the contemporary medical ethics movement can be traced to a growing concern in the mid–1960s with apparently widespread abuses of human rights in medical experimentation.[13] Responding to these concerns, the surgeon general of the United States issued a set of guidelines in 1966 for all research funded by the Public Health Service. These guidelines, the bulk of which are still in effect, required approval of all research on human subjects by a local review committee and procedures for obtaining written informed consent from all subjects of research prior to their participation in that research. Mild stuff by today's standards, these guidelines set the tone for much of what was to follow.

Like many social movements in the United States since World War II, medical ethics has moved in large part through—and, at times, been led by—the courts. Informed consent, in particular, is not only an ethical doctrine but also a legal one. The phrase itself originated in a 1957 California decision (*Salgo*) holding a physician liable for damages for withholding "any facts which are necessary to form the basis of an intelligent consent to the proposed treatment" and calling for "full disclosure of facts necessary to an informed consent."[14] The *Salgo* case was, moreover, only the first of a long string of such cases, with many extending the doctrine to require ever more exacting standards of disclosure. Since the 1960s, although with considerable variation from state to state, the doctrine of informed consent has been recognized in nearly every jurisdiction in the country.

The courts have also spoken loudly, if not always clearly, in matters con-

12. Consider, for example, Robert Veatch's claim in his introduction to *A Theory of Medical Ethics* (New York: Basic Books, 1981), p. 6: "In its extreme form, professional ethics can be seen as a highly particularistic ethic about which, in principle, only members of the profession can have knowledge. I shall examine the place we should give to such a professional ethic articulated by members of the profession and fully revealed only to those members. The only solution, I suggest, is to abandon the idea that an ethic for medicine can be based on a professionally articulated code."

13. Henry K. Beecher, "Ethics and Clinical Research," *New England Journal of Medicine* (1966) 174: 1354–60; Bradford Gray, *Human Subjects in Medical Experimentation* (New York: Wiley Interscience, 1975); Bernard Barber, John J. Lally, Julia Laughlin Makarushka, and Daniel Sullivan, *Research on Human Subjects* (New York: Russell Sage, 1973). For a history of these developments, see David Rothman, *Strangers at the Bedside* (New York: Basic Books, 1991).

14. For general discussions of informed consent as a legal doctrine, see Jay Katz, *The Silent World of Doctor and Patient* (New York: Free Press, 1984), chap. 3, and Ruth R. Faden and Tom L. Beauchamp, *A History and Theory of Informed Consent* (New York: Oxford University Press, 1986).

cerning termination of treatment. Although there is some evidence that physicians have long been prepared to withhold or withdraw treatments from terminally ill patients, the issues surrounding this practice burst into public consciousness only with the much celebrated 1976 Karen Quinlan case in New Jersey.[15] In the mere decade and a half since *Quinlan*, a remarkable body of case law has developed around the issues first raised in that case. With the United States Supreme Court's decision in the Cruzan case in June of 1990, there is now (albeit with some ambiguity) a "right to die" recognized by the country's highest court.[16]

Despite the importance of the courts, the success of medical ethics as a social movement is by no means limited to the law. Two national commissions—one dealing specifically with the protection of human subjects in biomedical research, the other having a broad mandate to examine ethical problems in medicine—have given quasi-official recognition to many of the insights of medical ethicists. Moreover, as a social movement, medical ethics has developed its own organizations, including most prominently the Hastings Center in New York and the Center for Bioethics at Georgetown University, but also "scores of other independent, academic, professional, and public interest associations, institutes, departments, and programs that have a major commitment to reflection, research, teaching, publishing and action in matters pertaining to bioethics." [17]

Not least, medical ethics has found a place within the core institutions of medicine itself. Articles on medical ethics, virtually unheard of before the mid–1960s, now appear routinely in the prestigious *New England Journal of Medicine* and the *Journal of the American Medical Association*. Courses on medical ethics, also rare before the mid–1960s, are now taught in virtually every medical school in the United States. And ethics committees, virtually unknown before the Quinlan case, now appear in various shapes and forms in growing numbers of hospitals.[18]

15. On the "prehistory" of termination of treatment, see Raymond S. Duff and A. G. M. Campbell, "Moral and Ethical Dilemmas in the Special Care Nursery," *New England Journal of Medicine* 289 (1973): 890–94. For a recent analysis of the Quinlan case, see Rothman, *Strangers*, chap. 11.

16. *Cruzan v. Director, Missouri Department of Health*, U.S. Supreme Court, 88–1503.

17. Fox, *Sociology of Medicine*, p. 227.

18. On the teaching of medical ethics, see Edmund D. Pellegrino and T. K. McIlhinney, *Teaching Ethics, the Humanities, and Human Values in Medical Schools: A Ten Year Overview* (Washington: Institute on Human Values, Society for Health and Human Values, 1981). On ethics committees, see Stuart J. Youngner, David L. Jackson, Claudia Coulton, Barbara Juknialis, and Era M. Smith, "A National Survey of Hospital Ethics Committees," *Critical Care Medicine* 11 (1983): 902–5; "Ethics Committees Double since '83: Survey," *Hospitals* 59 (1985): 60–64; S.

Although it would be a mistake to exaggerate the degree of consensus among ethicists or between ethicists and the courts or the federal government, one preoccupation has nonetheless dominated contemporary medical ethics since its origins. This is a preoccupation with patient autonomy or "self-determination," the empowerment of patients to make decisions for themselves.[19] It is a preoccupation which underlies the doctrine of informed consent and the effort, embodied in that doctrine, to allow patients greater participation in decisions bearing on their own health care. It is also a notion of autonomy that animated the Supreme Court's decision on termination of treatment in the Cruzan case. All of the justices save one (Scalia) acknowledged a patient's common law right to refuse treatment: the dissents in the divided court concerned only the best way to safeguard that right. But autonomy does not simply concern the patient. In practice, autonomy means autonomy from the discretion of physicians.

While the value placed on the patient's autonomy lies deep in American cultural and legal traditions, it is largely alien to medical traditions. Physicians, traditionally, have been more concerned with benevolence, with acting in what they construe to be the patient's best interest whether or not the patient himself or herself recognizes that interest. To be sure, academic medical ethicists have of late attempted to balance autonomy against other values with firmer bases in medical traditions.[20] While this new judiciousness represents something of a mellowing on the part of medical ethicists (and perhaps their partial absorption into the medical elite itself), the stress on self-determination remains the cutting edge of medical ethics as a social

---

Van McRay and Jeffrey Botkin, "Hospital Policy on Advance Directives," *Journal of the American Medical Association* 262 (1989): 2411–14.

19. For an influential discussion of autonomy, see President's Commission for the Study of Ethical Problems in Medicine and Biomedical and Behavioral Research, *Making Health Care Decisions*, vol. 1: *Report, the Ethical and Legal Implications of Informed Consent in the Patient-Practitioner Relationship* (Washington, DC: Government Printing Office, 1982), p. 44.

20. For a discussion of these attempts, see James Childress's reflections on the occasion of the Hastings Center's twentieth anniversary in "The Place of Autonomy in Bioethics," *Hastings Center Report*, January/February 1990, pp. 12–17. Since about 1980 there has also been an effort, concentrated particularly among physicians, to develop a somewhat different type of medical ethics, grounded self-consciously in medical traditions and medical practice. See, in particular, Mark Siegler, "Clinical Ethics and Clinical Medicine," *Archives of Internal Medicine* 139 (1979): 914–15; Albert R. Jonsen, Mark Siegler, and William J. Winslade, *Clinical Ethics: A Practical Approach to Ethical Decisions in Clinical Medicine* (New York: Macmillan, 1982); Edmund D. Pellegrino, "Clinical Ethics: Biomedical Ethics at the Bedside," *Journal of the American Medical Association* 260 (1988): 837–39. For a sympathetic critique of this "new casuistry," see John D. Arras, "Getting Down to Cases: The Revival of Casuistry in Bioethics," *Journal of Medicine and Philosophy* 16 (1991): 29–51.

movement. Physicians, after all, readily accept those values that are already theirs. But autonomy is different. Not only is it a value alien to medical traditions but it is a value that, when converted to rules and regulations, threatens physicians' authority.

The claim that medical ethics is an effort to regulate medicine does, however, call for considerable caution, for medical ethics is not the only attempt to regulate medicine and not even the most important. If I do not in this book discuss the efforts of the federal government or private employers to regulate medicine, I can plead only that there is an intellectual division of labor. My intention in this book is not to discuss all of the attempts to regulate, only those associated with medical ethics as a social movement.

Moreover, medical ethics itself is not an attempt to regulate all aspects of medicine. Medical ethics, at least as it has been conventionally understood in the United States, has had little to say about broad questions of health care financing. Although the origins of medical ethics as a social movement correspond roughly with the passage of Medicare and Medicaid, a self-identified ethical literature has contributed little to the continuing debates over how to eliminate remaining inequalities or how to control the costs of medical care. Nor has medical ethics addressed itself, except in the briefest passing, to the division of labor in medicine—to the "professional dominance" exercised by physicians over other health care workers. Rather, medical ethics has addressed itself primarily—indeed, almost exclusively—to clinical medicine. But this is no small matter, for medical ethics is an attempt to regulate the very practice of medicine and the everyday decisions—who to treat, in what ways, for what reasons—which only recently were the sole prerogative of physicians.

I do not mean to exaggerate the tension between medical ethics and physicians. Many courts and many ethicists have gone to great lengths both to understand and to make allowances for the traditions of medical practice. Their precepts are often intended to reflect, rather than change, what physicians actually do. At the same time, many physicians have greeted the rise of the medical ethics movement with enthusiasm, as welcome assistance in the often difficult decisions they are called on to make. I intend to treat as open questions whether or not other physicians resist the precepts of medical ethics, whether or not (and how) others turn medical ethics to their own purposes. I mean, for the moment, only to point in the general direction in which we are likely to find what tensions there are.

First, medical ethics substitutes principles and general rules for the case-by-case analysis that has long characterized medical practice. In some instances, ethicists have imported entire philosophical systems into medical practice. In others, they have been content to formulate a few basic principles and then apply them to specific situations. But in either instance the very effort to formulate general rules is fundamentally at odds with the physician's "conviction that cases are unique, that every patient represents his own unique set of problems that cannot be resolved by rigid application of some legalistically formulated rule."[21] Whatever the intellectual virtues of these two approaches—and arguments can be made for each—the difference goes well beyond conflicting styles of thought. For ethicists, lacking detailed knowledge of particular cases and rarely on hand when decisions are being made, the formulation of general principles provides the only means by which they can aspire to regulate clinical decisions. In contrast, for physicians, armed with a detailed knowledge of particular cases and constantly on hand, an insistence on case-by-case decision making is a means of maximizing their own discretion.

Second, medical ethics attempts to reformulate medical problems as moral, rather than technical, issues. Consider, for example, how Paul Ramsey, one the founders of medical ethics, introduces his classic study *The Patient as Person:*

This volume undertakes to examine some of the problems of medical ethics that are especially urgent in the present day. These are by no means technical problems on which only the expert (in this case, the physician) can have an opinion. They are rather the problems of human beings in situations in which medical care is needed.[22]

Just as physicians once attempted to convert moral issues to technical ones, medical ethicists attempt to convert technical issues to moral ones. And just as the physicians' conversion of issues to technical grounds helped them capture control of those issues, the medical ethicists' conversion of issues to moral grounds opens those issues back up to consideration beyond the medical profession itself. In looking for tensions between medical ethics and medical practice, we should not, then, look simply to different conceptions of right and wrong. Rather, the more fundamental tension is over the proper place of medical ethics and the proper place of technical medicine. If physicians resist medical ethics, they are less likely to do so by arguing that it is wrong than by arguing that it is irrelevant.

Somewhat more generally, I will suggest that there is now in medicine what might be called a "culture of rights"—a set of loose orientations incor-

21. Freidson, *Profession of Medicine*, pp. 44–45.
22. Paul Ramsey, *The Patient as Person* (New Haven: Yale University Press, 1970), p. xi.

porating many of the insights of medical ethics, including not least the value of patient autonomy. At the same time, however, there is also what might be called a "culture of the ward"—an even looser set of orientations derived from the direct experience of medical practice as well as from long medical tradition and directed far more to the expression of medical authority. These two cultures exist in uneasy tension. But the tension between them rarely centers on which culture physicians "belong" to. They belong to both. When physicians get down to actual cases, the tension is more often how, belonging to both, physicians continue to draw from each.

All this constitutes an agenda. None of the issues I have raised can be addressed in the abstract. Rather, they require detailed empirical investigation of ethics in practice in a particular place and at a particular time. My choice of a place to study medical ethics and the response of the medical profession to them was the intensive care unit of two hospitals. The time of my research was the late 1980s. And it is to a description of that time and those places that I must turn next.

2

Intensive Care

Of the other five patients, none could speak. Each suffered in the throes of some horrible, incurable, lingering disease that would almost certainly kill, usually involving major organs like heart, lung, liver, kidney, brain. The most pathetic was a man who had started with a pimple on his knee. . . . I saw his eyes fasten on me, a newcomer, someone who might bring a miracle, asking me to give him back his voice, his Saturday-afternoon game of squash, his piggyback rides under his kids. . . . I turned my head away. I never wanted to look into those mute eyes again.

He was not alone. Four more times I was shaken by the horror of ruined life. One after the other, totally immobilized, lungs run by respirators, hearts run by pacemakers, kidneys run by machines, brains run barely, if at all. It was terrible. . . .

I left. As I drove through the chill April rain, my mind stuck on the Unit. What about it had been so different?

Quintessence. That was it. The Unit was the quintessence. There, after all the sorting had been done, lay the closest representation, in living terms, of death. . . .

Berry asked me how it had been, and I told her that it had been different, high-powered, kind of like being part of the manned space program, but that it was also like being in a vegetable garden, only the vegetables were human.

Samuel Shem, *The House of God*[1]

When Albert DeLuca was admitted to the Intensive Care Unit at Countryside Hospital, his younger son, Edward, was shaken. "That was it. It was over. He was coughing up blood. He looked terrible, eyes were all flat and sunken in." Edward himself had been in intensive care earlier in the year, after an automobile accident, and had survived despite several weeks on a respirator. Still, despite his own experience—or, perhaps, because of it—he was frightened to see his father on a "breathing machine":

Scares me to see him on it. That's telling me that he can't breathe on his own. If it scares me to see it, I know if I was in that bed and it was hooked up to me, it would

1. Samuel Shem, *The House of God* (New York: Dell, 1978), pp. 326–30.

be scaring me. Because I know the only reason why that's in me is because I can't breathe on my own.

Donna George was frightened, too. A 50-year-old, Mrs. George had had asthma since childhood and had three times required hospitalization. But she had never been in an intensive care unit until she was admitted at Outerboro Hospital. To the doctors and nurses at Outerboro, hers was a routine case, easily managed with respiratory support and a likely success. But to Mrs. George herself, it was anything but routine. "I'd never been in an ICU," she told me after her discharge. "I never even visited anyone in ICU. That was the most horrifying experience I have ever been through in my whole life. I can't describe it. Don't ask me to. There's no describing it. . . . Most of the time I was in another world." She had, she said, spoken the day before to her son:

I was telling him, before I would ever go that route again, I said when I get out of here, I'm having the papers drawn up to that effect, that anything happens to me, I am dead serious, I am not going back to that ICU. Let me go. He said, no way, hell no. I said, just let me die with dignity. Don't put me through that kind of hell.

A physician, a patient's son, a patient: for each, intensive care held a special kind of horror—"the quintessence of death," a "kind of hell."

And yet . . .

Shem, who excoriates virtually every doctor and every rotation in a bitterly comic fictionalized account of his own internship, is comparatively gentle in his satire of intensive care. While Roy Basch, the novel's protagonist, can easily dismiss most medicine, the machine-like efficiency of intensive care is tempting and, so long as he is in the unit, absorbing: "It was difficult for me to say good-bye. I felt sad. I wanted to stay on. How do astronauts say good-bye?" [2] Edward DeLuca, though frightened, at least thought his father would get better care there. "So does my father. When he is in intensive care, he knows that he is going to be taken care of. When they move him out of intensive care down to the fourth floor or to the third floor or whatever, he is, like, 'Get me out of here.'" As frightening as intensive care may be, it is also reassuring. Even Mrs. George, all the while insisting she would never go back, acknowledged that she would not have survived without the unit's support.

2. Ibid, p. 356.

Outerboro and Countryside

With over one thousand beds, Outerboro Hospital is one of the half dozen largest hospitals in the state of New York. It is a teaching hospital, a primary affiliate of a New York City medical school. Situated in the Bronx, it serves a local population that is primarily poor, black, and Hispanic. But because of its excellent reputation, as well as the excellent reputation of the medical school with which it is affiliated, Outerboro also attracts a significant number of wealthy, private patients from the nearby Westchester suburbs.

Although significantly smaller than Outerboro, Countryside, with over six hundred beds, is one of the half dozen largest hospitals in Massachusetts. Like Outerboro, it is a teaching hospital, although not the primary affiliate of the Boston medical school with which it is associated. Situated on the border between city and country, it, too, draws patients from across the range of the class structure, although significantly fewer from among the very poor or the very wealthy than is the case at Outerboro.

At Outerboro and Countryside, as elsewhere, the intensive care unit is a hospital within the hospital. Not only is it more or less complete, with its own equipment and staff, but it is also separate. This separation from the rest of the hospital is, all at once, physical, organizational, and symbolic. Visitors and staff alike, at both Outerboro and Countryside, reach the unit through heavy double doors leading to a windowless corridor (longer at Outerboro, shorter at Countryside) that passes a nurses' station before coming to any of the patient beds. (Visitors must also pass signs alerting them to obtain permission before entering and then, with occasional exceptions, are limited to visits of usually no more than ten or fifteen minutes every two hours.)[3]

The Medical ICU at Outerboro had expanded in the two years just prior to my research from eight beds to twelve and, finally, to fourteen. Eight of the beds are arranged in two rows on an open ward; six beds are in private rooms along a separate corridor divided from the open ward by the nurses' station. The open ward is used for both men and women, the usual concern for modesty giving way to an apparent priority for genderless efficiency. The mixed Medical-Surgical ICU at Countryside has a twenty-four-bed capacity, although nursing shortages had typically limited effective capacity to sixteen or seventeen beds the year before, and to twenty-two beds while I was

---

3. On visiting more generally, see Stuart J. Youngner, Claudia Voulton, Robert Welton, Barbara Juknialis, and David L. Jackson, "ICU Visiting Policies," *Critical Care Medicine* 12 (1984): 606–9.

conducting my research. All but two of the beds are in private rooms. (The unit is also divided into three sections, each with its own nursing station, called "pods," a name that stuck after someone, during their construction, said they looked like spaceships.) The unit at Outerboro has its own small laboratory; the unit at Countryside has its own pharmacy. Both units have their own, specialized nursing staffs—with nearly forty nurses at Outerboro and over ninety at Countryside (including a few part-timers) providing one nurse for every two patients on each shift.

Although only a minority of intensive care units across the country have continuous medical coverage or a "functional" medical director,[4] Outerboro and Countryside have both, a pattern more frequent at larger hospitals. At Outerboro, three junior residents (two years out of medical school) and four interns (one year out of medical school) provide twenty-four-hour coverage. At Countryside, there are two separate teams of housestaff, one for the medical patients, the other for the surgical patients. The medical team—which, for purposes of comparison with Outerboro, was the focus of my research—consists of three interns and one senior resident (three years out of medical school). With the help of additional senior residents, who provide night coverage, the Countryside staff, like the Outerboro staff, provides round-the-clock coverage. Both units include "on-call rooms," where the housestaff can try to sleep (if they have not been called to answer an emergency) when they are on duty at night. At Outerboro, the housestaff is expected to remain in the unit at all times while on call, even eating their meals with food sent up from the cafeteria along with patients' trays. (The only exceptions—jokingly called "field trips" by the housestaff, in half-conscious reference to the rhythms and restrictions of life in junior high school—are that interns sometimes leave the unit to accompany patients to special procedures performed in other parts of the hospital.)

In both units the housestaff is supervised by senior ("attending") physicians. At Outerboro, two attendings round with the housestaff each morning, proceeding from bed to bed, discussing each case. Rounds, which begin at nine, usually last two to three hours. In addition, at least one attending is always available by phone. Most of the attendings rotate through the unit for a month at a time, although the unit director himself typically takes six such rotations in the course of a year. At Countryside, responsibility for the unit

4. Jack E. Zimmerman, "Administrative Structure of a Critical Care Unit," in Joseph E. Parillo and Stephen M. Ayres, eds., *Major Issues in Critical Care Medicine*, pp. 235–39 (Baltimore: William & Wilkins, 1984), and W. Vickrey Staughton and Vyatas Mickevicius, *Institutional Considerations Associated with the Operation of Intensive Care Units*, in ibid., pp. 255–64.

is shared among just three attendings, although each is assigned to the unit on a full-time basis. Each morning, one attending rounds with the medical housestaff and another with the surgical housestaff for roughly an hour. Rounds are repeated in the afternoon, and one attending is always available by phone.

Intensive care units are, above all, an organizational innovation. They are a means of concentrating staff to care for the most critically ill patients. "Critical care began," one observer has suggested, "when Florence Nightingale moved the more seriously ill but salvageable soldiers closer to the nurses' station."[5] Other observers have attributed the origins of intensive care to the special postoperative room instituted at Johns Hopkins in 1923 or to the special ward set up at Massachusetts General Hospital in 1942 to care for the victims of a fire at the Cocoanut Grove nightclub.[6] Yet, however long the traditions on which it can draw, intensive care did not become a convention of hospital care until the 1950s and 1960s. The heading "intensive care," for example, did not even appear in the *Cumulated Index* of medical articles until the 1955–59 edition. The Society of Critical Care Medicine was founded only in 1972, and an American Medical Association board began to certify specialists in intensive care only in 1986. In 1958, as Louise Russell has shown, only about one-quarter of even the largest community hospitals (those with more than three hundred beds) reported having an ICU. By 1976, "nearly all community hospitals with 200 beds or more reported one, not quite 90 percent of hospitals with 100 through 199 beds, and almost 50 percent of those with fewer beds."[7] Intensive care diffused from larger hospitals to smaller ones, from teaching hospitals to nonteaching ones, from private, nonprofit hospitals to private, for-profit and state or city hospitals.

In addition to proliferating among hospitals, intensive care has proliferated within hospitals. Where once one unit seemed sufficient, larger hospitals, particularly in the 1970s, began to establish several units that were more specialized. At Countryside, in addition to the mixed medical-surgical unit, there is a separate Cardiac Care Unit, a Neonatal Intensive Care Unit, and a Pediatric Intensive Care Unit. At Outerboro, in addition to the Medical ICU

5. Leigh Thompson, "Structure of Critical Care: An Overview," in Parillo and Ayres, eds., *Major Issues*, p. 225.

6. On the history of intensive care, see Mark Hilberman, "The Evolution of Intensive Care Units," *Critical Care Medicine* 3 (1975): 159–65; Henrich H. Bendixen and John M. Kinney, "History of Intensive Care," in John M. Kinney, Henrich H. Bendixen, and S. R. Powers, Jr., eds., *Manual of Surgical Intensive Care*, pp. 3–21 (Philadelphia: W. B. Saunders, 1977).

7. Louise Russell, *Technology in Hospitals: Medical Advances and Their Diffusion* (Washington, DC: Brookings Institution, 1979), p. 43.

and cardiac, neonatal, and pediatric units, there is a surgical unit and a neu-
rological unit. By the middle of the 1970s, intensive care accounted for more
than one of every twenty beds in acute care hospitals.

Intensive care serves the most acutely ill of hospital patients. The only
study I know of that systematically compares intensive care patients with
general ward patients—one conducted at the University Hospitals of Cleveland in 1983—found that ICU patients were approximately the same age (an
average of 59.3 years) as ward patients (58.2 years), were slightly more likely
to be men (49 percent to 43 percent), and were slightly more likely to be
nonwhite (51 percent to 48 percent).[8] While the demographic characteristics
of ICU patients were roughly similar to those of ward patients, their medical
conditions were not. Cardiovascular (48 percent to 30 percent), neurologic
(16 percent to 10 percent), and respiratory (27 percent to 19 percent) problems were far more common among intensive care patients than among ward
patients while gastrointestinal, renal, metabolic, and hematologic problems
were far more frequent among ward admissions (41 percent) than among
ICU patients (8 percent). Even more significantly, the medical staff at University Hospitals judged only 1 percent of the ward admissions to have less
than an even chance of surviving their hospital stay. In contrast, they judged
fully 40 percent of the ICU admissions to have less than an even chance.
Actual in-hospital death rates for ICU patients have been reported ranging
from 9 percent to 40 percent, with most of the variation accounted for by
differences in acuity of illness.[9]

At both Outerboro, in my own sample of 237 admissions, and at Countryside, in my sample of 117, admissions consisted primarily of patients in respiratory and cardiovascular distress. Beyond the broad similarities between
Outerboro and Countryside, there were, however, some specific differences.
My sample at Outerboro included thirty-six cancer patients (15 percent) and
forty-four patients with a primary diagnosis of a gastrointestinal bleed (19
percent). At Countryside, cancer patients made up only 8 percent of my
sample and patients with gastrointestinal bleeds, 7 percent. In contrast, 9
percent of admissions at Countryside were made up of suicide attempts,
compared to only 3 percent at Outerboro. AIDS patients accounted for 4
percent of admissions at both hospitals.

    8. Donna K. McLish, Andrea Russo, Cory Franklin, David L. Jackson, Wendy Lewan-
dowski, and Ingrid Alcover, "Profile of Medical ICU vs. Ward Patients in an Acute Care Hospital," *Critical Care Medicine* 13 (1985): 381–86.
    9. William A. Knaus, Elizabeth A. Draper, Douglas P. Wagner, and Jack E. Zimmerman,
"An Evaluation of Outcome from Intensive Care in Major Medical Centers," *Annals of Internal
Medicine* 1986 (104): 410–18.

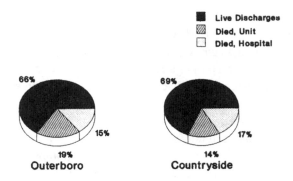

Figure 2.1. Intensive care death rates, percent of admissions.

Despite the differences in case mix, the outcomes of intensive care were roughly similar at Outerboro and Countryside. Nineteen percent of the patients admitted to the Outerboro Intensive Care Unit died without leaving the unit and an additional 15 percent without leaving the hospital. Fourteen percent of the Countryside patients died without leaving the unit, an additional 17 percent without leaving the hospital (see fig. 2.1). The severity of illness represented by the patients at Outerboro is probably among the highest of any ICU in the country. The severity of illness at Countryside, probably less than at Outerboro, is still probably considerably greater than is the case in most American ICUs.

Intensive care is not a technology. It is a place. But it is a place in which technology is applied daily to the most intractable of medical problems. Most generally, the principal roles of intensive care are "life-support of organ-system failure in critically ill patients or close monitoring of stable, noncritically ill patients in case the need for life support suddenly occurs." [10] More specifically, a 1983 conference sponsored by the National Institutes of Health identified the *minimum* technological capabilities of intensive care as including

A. Cardiopulmonary resuscitation
B. Airway management, including endotracheal intubation and assisted ventilation
C. Oxygen delivery systems and qualified respiratory therapists or registered nurses to deliver oxygen therapy

10. William A. Knaus, Elizabeth A. Draper, and Douglas P. Wagner, "The Use of Intensive Care: New Research Initiatives and Their Implications for National Health Policy," *Milbank Memorial Fund Quarterly* 61 (1983): 563.

D. Continual electrocardiograph monitoring

E. Emergency temporary cardiac pacing

F. Access to rapid and comprehensive laboratory services including but not limited to arterial blood gas analysis, electrolyte determinations, hemograms, measurement of cardiac enzymes, renal function studies, microbiologic studies, fluoroscopy, and other radiologic studies

G. Access to nutritional support services to advise on both enteral and parenteral nutritional techniques

H. Titrated therapeutic interventions with infusion pumps

I. Based on determination of the ICU patient composition, technological capability must be available to support therapeutic interventions that are commonly accepted medical practice. For example, an ICU that manages shock syndromes needs hemodynamic monitoring capability techniques to allow for the rational diagnostic categorization and subsequent therapy of patients with shock syndromes

J. Portable life-support equipment for use in patient transport, both within the hospital and for transfer[11]

Not only is each of these capabilities available at Outerboro and Countryside, many are routine. Heart rate and respiratory rate are monitored continuously for all but a few patients. Nearly one in every ten patients at both Outerboro and Countryside are supported in the unit after cardiopulmonary resuscitation, after they have stopped breathing or their hearts have stopped beating. Many are on dialysis, a process that does, artificially, the work of the kidney. Many more are on vasopressors, a powerful class of drugs used to maintain blood pressure. But it is endotracheal intubation—the placement of a tube through the trachea to assist with breathing in connection to a ventilator (and the treatment that both Edward DeLuca and Mrs. George found so frightening)—that is perhaps the most distinctive feature of intensive care. At Outerboro, well over half (56 percent) of the patients who pass through the ICU are intubated at some point in their stay. At Countryside, fully two-thirds (67 percent) are intubated. It is, then, in intensive care that men and women whose hearts have stopped are brought back to life, that machines breathe for those who cannot breathe for themselves, that patients who cannot eat are fed. Perhaps Lazarus is not quite raised from the dead, but it is in intensive care that the miracles of modern medical technology are reenacted routinely and methodically.

11. National Institutes of Health, *Consensus Development Conference Summary* 4 (1983), p. 7.

The Limits of Intensive Care

Miracles notwithstanding, intensive care has its disbelievers. Indeed, criticisms of intensive care—or, more precisely, of what goes on in intensive care—are almost as old as the units themselves. The most important of these criticisms, by virtue of its author's prominence and its place of publication, was a 1980 editorial published in the *New England Journal of Medicine* and written by the journal's editor, Arnold Relman.

First, according to Relman, patients and their visitors—like Mrs. George and Edward DeLuca—"often find the ICU to be a disturbing, even terrifying place."

Constant artificial light, ceaseless activity, frequent emergencies, and the ever-present threat of death create an atmosphere that can unnerve even the most phlegmatic of patients. Some are so sick that they are unaware of their surroundings or simply forget the experience, but for others the ICU is a nightmare remembered all too well.[12]

Second, according to Relman, intensive care units are not only frightening. "They are terribly expensive."[13] By most estimates a day in intensive care costs three to four times as much as a day spent elsewhere in the hospital.[14] As a result, the roughly 5 percent of the in-hospital patient population found in ICUs consumes between 15 and 20 percent of all hospital costs, a total approaching 1 percent of the entire Gross National Product. Moreover, intensive care may drain resources from other parts of the hospital. The concentration of housestaff and attendings in intensive care diverts them from other parts of the hospital and from primary care. The concentration of skilled nurses may result (in language that is not Relman's) in a reduction of skills among nurses on general floors.

Third, and most important, Relman suggested that the "cost and psychological stress of ICU treatment would be justifiable if such units were known

12. Arnold Relman, "Intensive Care Units: Who Needs Them?" *New England Journal of Medicine* 302 (1980): 965.
13. Ibid.
14. See, for example, Edward W. Campion, Albert G. Mulley, Richard L. Goldstein, G. Otto Barnett, and George E. Thibault, "Medical Intensive Care for the Elderly: A Study of Current Use, Costs, and Outcomes," *Journal of the American Medical Association* 246 (1981): 2052–56; Mark R. Chassin, "Costs and Outcomes of Medical Intensive Care," *Medical Care* 20 (1982): 165–79; Jeffrey R. Parno, Daniel Teres, Stanley Lemeshow, and Richard B. Brown, "Hospital Charges and Long-Term Survival of ICU versus Non-ICU Patients," *Critical Care Medicine* 10 (1982): 569–74. Even controlling for severity of illness, intensive care units remain significantly more expensive than other parts of the hospital. Claudia Coulton, Donna McLish, Harvey Doremus, Stephen Powell, Stephen Smookler, and David L. Jackson, "Implications of DRG payments for Medical Intensive Care," *Medical Care* 23 (1985): 977–85.

to reduce mortality and morbidity from levels achievable with less costly and intensive modes of hospital care." But, Relman continued, "there have been no prospective, randomized, controlled trials to supply such data."[15] Like many medical treatments, the diffusion of intensive care (and particularly cardiac care units) seems to have depended more on faith in science than on scientific evidence itself.

This is not an unusual pattern in American medicine. Although physicians draw on scientific research, they are not themselves scientists but clinicians. Their interest is not in the formulation of general principles but in the application of those principles to particular cases. They are, by consequence, prepared to take up any treatment that they think makes good sense, even if they do not have evidence beyond their own experience and intuition. The widespread resort to coronary artery bypass surgery, for example, preceded convincing evidence that it effectively reduced myocardial infarctions and continued at a near breakneck pace even despite later evidence that it was sometimes ineffective.

In the case of intensive care, the rapidity of its diffusion seems to have been encouraged by a number of considerations more or less independent of its effectiveness. As an organizational innovation, intensive care seemed to make sense as a management tool and as an answer to the recurring nursing shortages characteristic of the post–World War II American labor force. As a set of technologies designed for the acutely ill, it fit in comfortably with a long-standing emphasis in American medicine on cure rather than prevention, with a focus on "heroics" rather than primary care.[16]

Intensive care is, then, perhaps the ultimate expression of what Paul Ramsey has called the "physician's search for exquisite triumphs over death in a sort of salvation by works."[17] Although somewhere between 60 and 90 percent of ICU patients survive their hospital stay, mortality is much higher for some specific conditions. For example, death rates reach as high as 60 percent among patients in respiratory failure who require ventilator support for

15. Relman, "Intensive Care Units," p. 966.
16. In *The Second Sickness* (New York: Free Press, 1983) Howard Waitzkin has drawn far-reaching conclusions from the lack of convincing data on the effectiveness of intensive care. According to Waitzkin, one of the most strident critics of intensive care, the rapid diffusion of special care units can be attributed to the influence of pharmaceutical and medical equipment companies eager to find new product markets. Although Waitzkin is certainly right that companies like Werner-Lambert have been interested parties in—and avid boosters of—the growth of intensive care, he assigns them altogether too much influence. The rise of intensive care does not need a special explanation. It is entirely in keeping with the general pattern of American medicine.
17. Paul Ramsey, *The Patient as Person* (New Haven: Yale University Press, 1970), p. 115.

more than three days. Among patients with both respiratory failure requiring ventilator support and kidney failure, the death rate approaches 80 or 90 percent.[18] And at least one study suggests that "survival becomes unprecedented when three or more organ system failures persist for more than 48 hours."[19]

Moreover, it is often the most acutely ill patients, with the poorest chance of survival, who linger longest in the unit and at greatest cost. One study found that "nonsurvivors" of intensive care incurred hospital charges nearly twice as high as survivors and averaged 5.3 days in the unit compared to 3.3 for survivors.[20] Of the seventy-nine patients in my sample who died at Outerboro, the average length of stay in the unit was 9.0 days, compared to 5.3 for those who survived their hospital stay. At Countryside, the average length of stay for those who died was 4.9 days, compared to 3.7 for those who survived (see fig. 2.2). As a result, patients who will die without leaving the hospital make up a far higher proportion of patients in the unit at any given time than they do of patients admitted to the unit. At both Countryside (20.2 percent) and Outerboro (20.3 percent), one-fifth of the beds are occupied by patients who will die without leaving the unit. Another quarter (28.0 percent) of the patients in the Countryside unit at any given time and nearly a third (32.6 percent) of the Outerboro patients will die without leaving the hospital (see fig. 2.3).

Ethics and Intensive Care

Filled with patients and staff who find it terrifying, consuming an enormous share of hospital resources, treating patients whose eventual death is often a foregone conclusion, intensive care is a virtual laboratory for the exploration of some of the most central issues in contemporary medical ethics. Part I of this book addresses the fate of the doctor-patient relationship in intensive care, the forces pushing toward a construction of that relationship in narrowly technical terms stripped of moral content, and the forces pushing toward a reconstruction of that relationship around emergent notions of patients' rights. Part II turns to two more conventional issues in medical ethics,

18. Thomas A. Raffin, Joel N. Shurkin, and Wharton Sinkler, *Intensive Care* (New York: W. H. Freeman, 1989), p. 14.

19. William A. Knaus, Elizabeth A. Draper, and Douglas P. Wagner, "Evaluating Medical Surgical Intensive Care Units," in Parillo, ed., *Major Issues*, p. 40.

20. Allan S. Detsky, Steven C. Stricker, Albert G. Mulley, and George E. Thibault, "Prognosis, Survival, and the Expenditure of Hospital Resources for Patients in an Intensive Care Unit," *New England Journal of Medicine* 305 (1981): 667–72.

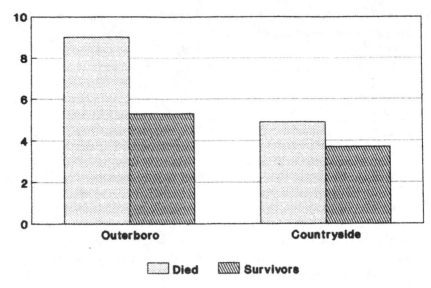

Figure 2.2. Length of stay in days, by hospital discharge status.

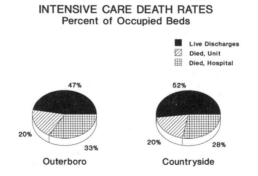

Figure 2.3. Intensive care death rates, percent of occupied beds.

although in an unconventional way. Chapters 8–13 address decisions to withhold treatment from terminally ill patients, but with an emphasis on how and why those decisions are in fact made rather than on how they should be made. Chapter 14 discusses triage, the procedures by which physicians decide who should receive treatment in intensive care and who should not, and the social factors influencing those decisions.

Doctors and Medical Ethics

The history of intensive care, its technical capabilities, and the sometimes questionable effectiveness of its interventions set an agenda common to both Outerboro and Countryside. But, while the similarities between the two units are probably greater than any differences, the responses of the units are not always the same. I cannot claim any great foresight in my choice of research sites. But I had the good fortune, largely by accident, to conduct my research in two units characterized by significantly different emphases in their response to common problems.

There were differences in behavior. In general, the Countryside physicians were more concerned with triage—with keeping beds available for those patients who would benefit from them most—than were the Outerboro physicians. In contrast, the Outerboro physicians were somewhat more insistent than those at Countryside on pursuing every therapeutic possibility, even for patients in apparently terminal stages of illness. Thus, the Countryside physicians were somewhat quicker to withhold or withdraw treatment than were those at Outerboro. While the average length of a unit stay was, in general, longer at Outerboro than at Countryside, the difference was considerably larger among those who died without leaving the hospital (9.0 days to 4.9 days) than among those who survived (5.3 days to 3.7).[21]

There was also a difference in style. At Outerboro, issues relevant to medical ethics, although discussed often, were a matter many attending physicians thought better left to doctors, with as little "outside interference" as possible. "I think most of the people who write" medical ethics, one Outerboro attending told me, "have very little training and have very little insight as to what is going on. . . . I am very comfortable with the way I make decisions, and I let myself be guided by something internal what I think is right and what I think is humane." In contrast, the attendings at Countryside were somewhat more open to the influence of philosophy, law, and the social sciences. Although complaints about the intrusions of these disciplines into the domain of physicians could be heard at Countryside as well as at Outerboro, at Countryside they were more readily acknowledged as legitimate influences on decisions that demanded the physicians' attention. The director of

---

21. Calculated from a sample of discharges (233 at Outerboro, 117 at Countryside), the point is even stronger. The average length of unit stay for seventy-six hospital survivors in this sample at Countryside is 4.4 days; at Outerboro, at 4.8 days (n = 137), it is only slightly higher. In contrast, the average length of stay is more than double for the Outerboro nonsurvivors (n = 92) than for the Countryside nonsurvivors (n = 40), 10.2 days to 4.7.

the unit, for example, included sections on both law and ethics in courses he taught on hospital administration at a nearby college and is an active participant in the hospital's Ethics Committee, a committee which includes lay people as well as physicians. This is not to say that the Outerboro physicians failed to act ethically or that the Countryside physicians succeeded in acting ethically. To the contrary, I was impressed, time and time again, by the high standards to which the physicians at both hospitals held themselves. It is only to say that at Outerboro the physicians were guided, somewhat more than at Countryside, "by something internal," internal to themselves as individuals and internal to themselves as members of the medical profession.

I cannot claim that Outerboro and Countryside are representative of intensive care units, or even of intensive care units in large teaching hospitals. There are far too many variations in administrative arrangements, patient populations, and unit policies for any two units to represent very much more than themselves. Moreover, even at the two hospitals I studied, my own research is very much time bound. I conducted the bulk of my research at Outerboro between 1985 and 1987 and the bulk of my research at Countryside in 1989. However, these qualifications notwithstanding, the problems that physicians, nurses, patients, and families faced at Outerboro and Countryside during the time I studied them are very general ones. If Outerboro and Countryside tell us very little about the distribution of responses to those problems, they will, I hope, tell us a good deal about the range of responses and the social logic underlying them.

My research included regular attendance at morning rounds at Outerboro in six separate sequences of nineteen days each and regular attendance at morning and afternoon rounds at Countryside in three separate sequences, also of nineteen days each. My notes, taken during rounds, fill over fifty bound notebooks. In addition, I conducted formal interviews with residents and interns, attendings, nurses, and (with the help of Jonathan Sharpe) patients at Outerboro. At Countryside, in addition to residents and interns, attendings, nurses, and patients, I was also able to interview a number of patients' families. At both hospitals, I reviewed charts and records and, most important, generally hung out, often sitting in the doctor's lounge, listening to and chatting with whoever had the time and tolerance to do so. (For those who are interested, I have included a more detailed discussion of my methods in an appendix.) In reporting cases, I have taken the liberty of editing my field notes in the interest of clarity but material included in quotation marks is verbatim, taken either from my field notes or from transcriptions of interviews.

Patients and their families, nurses, and physicians are identified only by pseudonyms, as are "Outerboro" and "Countryside" themselves. In a number of instances, I have altered or omitted details in order to protect confidentiality. Despite these occasional distortions, I have chosen to assign names because omitting them altogether would have distorted matters even more. I have also followed a pattern of referring to most physicians by first name and most patients by last name—reproducing the style of address characteristic of the physicians themselves. Although decisions in intensive care are shaped, in part, by impersonal forces, they are also shaped, especially in specific cases, by the idiosyncrasies of individuals. Intensive care is peopled. Although many different physicians, nurses, patients, and family members appear on the pages that follow, six reappear sufficiently frequently to warrant their introduction in advance: Dennis, the director of Outerboro's Intensive Care Unit; Mark, a frequent attending physician at Outerboro; John, the director of intensive care at Countryside; Ken, the director of the Medical Service in Countryside's ICU; Scranton Haskell, an elderly cancer patient whose long stay in the ICU was the occasion for some of the most extended discussions of medical ethics at Outerboro; and Kelly Connors, a twenty-year-old whose long stay in the Countryside ICU was the occasion for many of the most extended discussions of medical ethics in that hospital.

Part 1

THE MORAL ORDER OF
INTENSIVE CARE

Contemporary medicine, if we are to believe its critics, is impersonal and bureaucratic. Treatment consists of discrete interventions with little attention to the patient as a whole person—someone with hopes and fears as well as a disease, someone living in a distinctive social setting with its own special stresses and problems. Doctors, we are told, particularly in hospital settings, barely know their patients and show little interest in coming to know them better. Under the spell of technology and scientific medicine, doctors have lost interest in the art of medicine—particularly in the talk, sometimes soothing, sometimes coaxing, that once made the doctor-patient relationship itself a critical part of the therapeutic process.[1] All this is undoubtedly true and, perhaps, nowhere so much as in intensive care. But it is also, at best, partial.

First, the impersonality of medicine, so thoroughly excoriated by medicine's critics, brings with it another development those very same critics are more likely to welcome. The disappearance of an orientation to the patient as a person goes hand in hand with the disappearance of a sometimes oppressive moralizing. Certainly, sociologists and historians have been quick to point out that physicians' moral judgments are rife with class and ethnic bias and often mask what is, in effect, an agenda of social control.[2] But moral judgments—judgments that some patients are more or less "worthy" of

1. See, among many others, Stanley Reiser, *Medicine and the Reign of Technology* (New York: Cambridge University Press, 1979); Edward Shorter, *Bedside Manners* (New York: Simon & Schuster, 1985); Terry Mizrahi, *Getting Rid of Patients* (New Brunswick, NJ: Rutgers University Press, 1986).
2. See, again among many others, Morris Vogel, *The Invention of the Modern Hospital* (Chicago: University of Chicago Press, 1980); David Rosner, *A Once Charitable Enterprise* (Princeton: Princeton University Press, 1987); and Charles Rosenberg, *The Care of Strangers* (New York: Basic Books, 1987), for historical material. See David Sudnow, *Passing On: The Social Organiza-*

29

medical care than others, that "appropriate" treatment may demand reforming character as well as administering drugs or procedures—require at least
a rudimentary knowledge of and interest in the patient's social situation and
background. Yet, at least in intensive care, both this knowledge and this interest are lacking. If contemporary medicine is less personal, it is also more
tolerant. It is prepared to offer help not only to the solid citizen or the blameless victim but also to those of more often questioned character. It is prepared to treat the drug user, the drinker, the diabetic who fails to take her
insulin, the man with kidney disease who misses his appointments for dialysis, with the same principled indifference that is, in other circumstances,
a source of strident criticism.

Second, if the close personal relationship between doctor and patient has
become a thing of the past (if indeed it ever existed at all), it has been replaced by a relationship organized around different principles. In particular,
in the absence of a personal relationship—in the absence, as it were, of
trust—the doctor-patient relationship has been reorganized around principles of patients' rights. Most important, the doctrine of "informed consent" has created a new role for patients as participants in their own care.[3]
To be sure, even in the age of informed consent, and particularly in intensive
care, contemporary medicine is dominated by what doctors do to patients
rather than by what patients do for themselves. What is different is that patients are now called on to participate in deciding what it is that doctors will
do to them.

Chapters 3 (on patients), 4 (on doctors), and 5 (on nurses) are about the
impersonality of intensive care medicine although each introduces a slight
twist on conventional criticisms of contemporary medicine. Chapter 6 discusses rights and the ways in which an emphasis on them emerges out of the
very impersonality of intensive care. Chapter 7 returns to patients and how
they, along with their families, are oriented to the exercise of rights.

---

tion of Dying (Englewood Cliffs, NJ: Prentice Hall, 1967), for an influential sociological statement.

3. See, for example, Michael Betz and Lenahan O'Connell, "The Changing Doctor-Patient
Relationship and the Rise in Concern for Accountability," *Social Problems* 31 (1983): 84–95; Jay
Katz, *The Silent World of Doctor and Patient* (New York: Free Press, 1984); Ruth R. Faden and
Tom L. Beauchamp, *A History and Theory of Informed Consent* (New York: Oxford University
Press, 1986).

3

The Patient

Personhood, we might like to think, is something inherent in each of us. Perhaps, in some philosophic sense, it is. But personhood, in another sense, is also something that must be achieved and guarded. It consists of the ability to participate in (and, to some degree, direct) the events surrounding our own lives, the ability to express an identity and (good or bad) a moral character. Personhood, in this sense, is not inherent but something that becomes manifest only in social situations. Personhood, in this sense, is something that may be denied by illness. It may also be denied by those who treat illness.[1]

"A Little Bit of a Science Project"

In their now classic article "The Basic Models of the Doctor-Patient Relationship," Thomas Szasz and Marc Hollander argue that the degree to which medical care involves the patient as a participant in his or her own treatment depends heavily on the quality of illness.[2] In cases of chronic illness (ranging from diabetes to psychoneuroses), they argue, the very "notions of disease and health lose most of their relevance" and are replaced by concepts of behavior and adaptation.[3] By consequence, the character of the patient—the patient's willingness to reform long-held patterns of behavior, to accommodate to an often difficult medical regimen—becomes an essential part of treatment. In contrast, in cases of acute disease, which make up much of the

1. This formulation draws heavily, albeit somewhat indirectly, on the work of Erving Goffman. See, in particular, his *Stigma: Notes on the Management of Spoiled Identity* (Englewood Cliffs, NJ: Prentice Hall, 1963).
2. Thomas Szasz and Marc Hollander, "Basic Models of the Doctor-Patient Relationship," *Archives in Internal Medicine* 97 (1956): 585–92. There is an ambiguity in the Szasz and Hollander article on whether the basic models are meant as models of appropriate behavior or models of actual behavior. I have treated them here as models of actual behavior.
3. Ibid., p. 589.

practice of contemporary hospital medicine, the notion of disease consists of specific signs and symptoms while treatment consists primarily of what the doctor does to the patient. The patient may be asked to cooperate with a specific regimen, to follow "doctor's orders," but the demands on the patient typically fall far short of a total reorganization of a way of life. Finally, in cases in which the patient is unconscious, whether in a coma or during surgery, the patient is entirely passive. Diagnosis and treatment alike, Szasz and Hollander argue, take place "irrespective of the patient's contribution."[4] Treatment consists entirely of what the doctor does to the patient, and the patient's participation is beside the point.

The bearing of all this on the matters at hand is that it is the third model of the doctor-patient relationship that predominates in intensive care. "In the unit," one resident explained, "it is a little bit of a science project. . . . That's basically what people are reduced to. It's blood pressure, temperature, respirations, and their cardiogram." In this sense, if we are to follow Szasz and Hollander, the patient vanishes in intensive care—not, of course, as an object of treatment but, in any meaningful sense, as a participant.

In other settings, diagnosis begins as a doctor takes a patient's history. The taking of a history may not exactly make the patient a coparticipant in medical care, but it is a process in which the character of the patient is expressed, in which the patient's own narrative is the starting point for medical treatment. In intensive care, however, doctors and nurses are often called on to treat patients who cannot give histories. There are extreme cases, as one resident explained: "At least one of those a month, an unknown male found on the street by EMS [Emergency Medical Service], with an overdose or unresponsive. There's no history. . . . Basically you are depending on the exam and the numbers, and there's no human interaction at all." Even when physicians and nurses do know a patient's history, at least in basic outline, that history often becomes little more than a secondary source, replaced by the objective measures of laboratory-generated data. "Good doctors never look at the history of the patient," Ken, the Countryside unit's medical director, explained one day during rounds. "They just look at the numbers." Even the physical exam, the literal laying on of hands that implies at very least an acknowledgement of the patient's physical presence, becomes less important in the setting of intensive care. "I don't talk to patients," Ken insisted on another day, after a woman's private physician reported that the patient had said she was feeling fine. "This is the patient," the private physician an-

4. Ibid., p. 586.

swered, perhaps only half joking as he held up the flow sheet that listed the woman's laboratory values. An Outerboro resident explained:

I think you don't have to look at a patient here, basically. You don't have to really examine a patient. . . . Someone has a PA [pulmonary artery] line in, you don't have to listen to their lungs. . . . In that respect, with technology you don't have to deal with a patient, examine a patient. The numbers, I feel, they are more reliable.

And as another put it, in a striking image in which the irrelevance of the patient's personhood becomes altogether apparent, "In a way it's almost like veterinary medicine."

Of the 237 patients whose admissions I observed at Outerboro, 35 (15 percent) were admitted with, in the language of the unit, "no mental status"—unable to speak and unresponsive to voice, apparently unaware of place or person.[5] Of 111 admissions at Countryside, 19 (17 percent) were unresponsive. These are patients who cannot, in any sense, participate in their own care. To the doctors and nurses who work in the unit, they are, by result of the very conditions that bring them to the unit, objects of treatment. An additional 65 patients at Outerboro (27 percent) and 29 patients at Countryside (26 percent) entered the unit stuporous or lethargic, able (in some cases) to speak and respond but usually unaware of where they were, let alone why (see fig. 3.1).

Moreover, to the conditions the ICU is intended to treat are added the character of the treatments themselves. At Outerboro and Countryside, as at most hospitals, a basic service of intensive care is to support patients in respiratory distress, whether from pneumonia, severe asthma, heart disorders,

	Outerboro		Countryside	
No Mental Status	15%	(n = 35)	17	(19)
Stuporous	27	(65)	26	(29)
Alert	58	(137)	57	(63)
Intubated	18	(43)	28	(31)
Not Intubated	40	(94)	29	(32)
Total	100	(237)	100	(111)

Figure 3.1. Mental status of ICU patients.

5. The concept of "no mental status," as it is used at Outerboro and elsewhere, is not limited to patients who are "brain dead," a relatively rare condition. Patients are said to have "no mental status" when they are unresponsive except to pain. In general, "no mental status" refers to patients who are unable to take part in any meaningful human interaction.

or any number of other conditions. This is done by supporting the patient with a mechanical respirator, a process which usually requires "intubation," the placement of a tube leading from the respirator through the patient's nose or mouth and then through the esophagus. Intubation is not only painful but also prevents the patient from speaking. An intubated patient cannot give a history, cannot register complaints, cannot communicate, except by shakes of the head and laboriously written notes—and this only when the sedatives used to control the pain of the process are not too heavy.[6] Thus, many of the patients who enter the unit alert are soon faced with an added handicap to their participation in their own care. Of the 137 patients who entered the Outerboro unit alert, 43 (31 percent of the alert patients, 18 percent of all patients) were intubated within twenty-four hours of admission. Of the 63 patients who entered the Countryside unit alert, 31 (49 percent of the alert patients, 28 percent of all patients) were intubated within twenty-four hours of admission. In all, then, only 94 of the 237 (40 percent) of the Outerboro patients and 32 of the 111 (29 percent) Countryside patients whose admission I observed were neither stuporous nor intubated.

Yet even these figures understate the degree to which intensive care is occupied by unresponsive patients. Patients who are neither stuporous nor intubated are healthier than those who are. As a result, their ICU stay is usually shorter (an average of 3.7 days, compared to 8.3 days for those who were intubated or not alert at Outerboro; 1.6 days compared to 4.5 at Countryside). Put a little differently, patients who entered the unit alert and who were not quickly intubated accounted for less than one-quarter of all patient days in the unit at Outerboro and less than one-seventh at Countryside. Moreover, many patients decline over the course of their ICU stay. The result, then, is often a unit caring almost entirely for unresponsive patients.

Consider one day at Outerboro. Seven of the eight beds in the open ward were full.

Bed 1: Irving Krickstein had been stuporous on admission, five days earlier, and unresponsive to questions. He was intubated and sedated soon after his admission. Although the ICU staff had lightened up on his sedation, he was still intubated and "doing badly" when asked to answer questions.
Bed 2: Empty.

6. See Ingered Bergbom-Engberg and Hengo Haljame, "Patient Experiences during Respirator Treatment—Reason for Intermittent Positive-Pressure Ventilation Treatment and Patient Awareness in the Intensive Care Unit," *Critical Care Medicine* 17 (1989): 22–25.

Bed 3: Peter Edwards had been intubated and sedated on admission, nine days earlier. Although one of the interns described him as "clear" when she reduced his sedation, he was still intubated.

Bed 4: Jack Reilly, intubated early in his ICU stay, had been in the unit for forty-eight days. Initially, according to a note in the chart, he had been "very agitated" but, for the last month, had been "minimally responsive— even to needle sticks." According to one of the residents, he did squeeze his wife's hand when she visited but was otherwise unresponsive.

Bed 5: The only new admission of the day was an unidentified, unresponsive man who had been brought to the hospital from a men's shelter by Emergency Medical Service. "The only history we got," an intern explained during his presentation, "was from his chest, which showed multiple surgery."

Bed 6: Edith Green had been brought to the hospital unresponsive "except to deep pain" and had remained so for thirteen days.

Bed 7: Max Kohler had been admitted with slurred speech. He had been intubated and sedated since his admission five days earlier.

Bed 8: Lotte Baer, in her fourth day in the ICU, was the only patient on the ward who was alert and oriented.

All six of the beds in the back section of the unit were full:

Bed 9: Max Rosenberg had been brought to the hospital with an "altered mental status" and was intubated in the Emergency Room even before his admission to the ICU. Although his mental status had improved over the course of his five-day stay and he was now "totally there," he had not responded to attempts to wean him from the respirator and remained intubated.

Bed 10: Alberto Rodriguez had been intubated on the second of his seven days in the ICU. Over the course of the week, his alertness had waxed and waned. He was now alert but still intubated.

Bed 11: Angel Santiago had been brought to the unit the day before in a diabetic coma. "He was tubed within ten minutes of coming up," one intern explained, "so we don't have much history." Although the same intern described Santiago's mental status as now improved, he remained intubated and unresponsive to commands to open and close his eyes.

Bed 12: Georgia Johnson had been admitted to the unit fifty-six days earlier following a respiratory arrest and was later diagnosed as having fatal esophageal cancer. Intubated even before her ICU admission, she was now alert and able to sit up in a chair but unable to speak and able to communicate at all only with great difficulty through a few signs.

Bed 13: Allan Lerner had been admitted to the unit the same day as Georgia Johnson and also intubated immediately for the chronic lung disease that would result in his death. In addition to his intubation, he had been "morbidly depressed" even before his admission. It was not clear to the ICU staff how much he understood, although one of the nurses did report that he squeezed her hand in response to questions.

Bed 14: Audrey Roland had been admitted to the unit fifteen days earlier, intubated and sedated a few days later. Although alert, the frequent notes she wrote showed little understanding that she was in a hospital.

Such patients are poor candidates for participation in their own care.

"There can be," one Outerboro resident insisted, "a very nice relationship . . . if you have an awake and alert patient who's not intubated." But, he quickly acknowledged, this is not usually the case.

The relationship with the patient . . . who comes in comatose and debilitated, unable to speak for themselves or respond to you . . . is a difficult one. You're often left with a sense of, What am I doing here? That is, the patient has been dehumanized, not by any act of people but just by the disease that's happened. Here we are with a mass of protoplasm.

"They have names," another resident added, "but we speak of the patient in that bed with this problem. Because a lot of people are intubated, they can't talk. And so you've got to just deal with them not as a person but as a problem, a set of numbers and dynamics. We're not dealing with a walking, talking person."

Good Medicine

Only the most determined sociological reductionist would deny the brute force of disease and disability in denying ICU patients their personhood. But if it is physiology that denies personhood to many ICU patients, it is a distinctive notion of what constitutes good medicine that denies personhood to the rest. Intensive care, in particular, is organized around a notion that medicine at its best—at its most heroic, its purest—is about physiology and physiology alone.[7]

7. For dicussions of intensive care that proceed along similar lines, see Stuart J. Youngner, ed., *Human Values in Critical Care Medicine* (New York: Praeger, 1986); Joel E. Frader and

The mission of intensive care is, explicitly and without apology, to deal with medical crises. "The unit," according to one Outerboro resident,

is really a place to get people over a kind of medical disaster. It's a place you just try to get them out of alive, and you don't worry about [other things]. You treat the immediate problem. You don't necessarily deal with the other underlying chronic problems or what is this person going to do when they go home or any of that stuff. You deal with the acute problem.

Intensive care addresses acute physiological problems. Other considerations are simply crowded out. "All we care about in the unit," a Countryside resident stressed, echoing the sentiments of his counterpart at Outerboro, "is making sure somebody is alive."

If, in other settings, as medicine's critics complain, the patient is reduced to a disease, in intensive care physicians may focus on a particular physiological process in which even the underlying disease is forgotten. "Usually," an Outerboro resident explained, the reason a patient is in the unit "is because of an infection superimposed [on something else] or a GI [gastrointestinal] bleed superimposed [on something else]. . . . We try and stop that. But the underlying problem often doesn't make any difference." Thus, the ICU physicians treat the respiratory distress that results from cancer but often not the cancer itself; they treat the gastrointestinal bleed that results from underlying liver disease but not the liver disease itself.

If ICU physicians sometimes ignore underlying disease in favor of treating immediate problems, they are even less attentive to the broader context of that disease. To be sure, even in the abbreviated histories characteristic of intensive care, some physicians remain acutely aware of social, environmental, and emotional components in the etiology of disease. In discussing the ethnically diverse patients at Outerboro, most housestaff, even in the ICU, routinely mention at least something about the patient's social background as a possible diagnostic clue. At both hospitals, housestaff often mention something about the patient's living situation and, where relevant, histories of drug use, alcohol use, and cigarette smoking as well as occupational hazards to which a patient might have been exposed. Yet, however interested in such factors as explanations of the origins of disease, physicians in the ICU remain indifferent to them in its treatment. "When they get to the floor," a Countryside resident explained, drawing a contrast with the unit, "then you start with, do they have nurses at home to take care of them, are they getting

Charles L. Bosk, "Patient Talk at Intensive Care Unit Rounds," *Social Science and Medicine* 15 (1981): 267–74; Renee R. Anspach, "Notes on the Sociology of Medical Discourse: The Language of Case Presentation," *Journal of Health and Social Behavior* 29 (1988): 357–75.

home oxygen. . . . Here we do what we have to do [to] get the patient better."
With his characteristic bluntness Ken, the unit's medical director, drove
home a similar point when one of the interns raised questions about psycho-
genic components in the treatment of a 72-year-old woman who had been
brought to the unit pulseless: "We don't talk about psychiatric disorders
here." Put simply, it is specific, discrete treatments, abstracted from any social or emotional context, that constitute good medicine in intensive care.
The physician's job, at least as physicians themselves understand it, is to treat
acute physiological conditions and little else.

The narrowing of the ICU physicians' interest is perhaps most apparent
in the suicide attempts they are occasionally called on to treat. Consider, for
example, the case of Matt Flowers, an 18-year-old with a severe learning
disability, seriously depressed for two months, and admitted to the Outerboro ICU after having taken an overdose of drugs. While the presentation of
Flowers's case made due reference to emotional strains, the medical staff
were quick to reassert their primary focus. The "major concern," the intern
in charge of the case explained, "is damage to the liver." And the "only mys-
terious thing about him," an attending added, "is why he's still asleep." That
evening Flowers's sister brought in his suicide note, written in a childish
scrawl. The next day it was exhibited at rounds: "Dear Mommy, I love you.
I don't want to rember [*sic*] no one or anything at all." Seeing the note, one
resident said simply, "It's very sad." But the attending physician was quick
to remind him of the proper focus: "This suggests there's impaired functioning."

None of this is to say that the ICU physicians and nurses are indifferent
to human suffering. They are not. Indeed, there are many instances of small
kindnesses. The ICU nurses and physicians constantly reassure patients,
sometimes even when they are not sure the patients understand, but just on
the off chance that they might. A nurse goes out of her way to tie a bow in
the hair of a depressed, elderly woman. For the rare patient who lingers
in the ICU for many days, alert and conscious, the physicians and nurses
often provide a few extras—making sure, for example, that such a patient
has a television or radio (not standard in the Outerboro unit) or, at Countryside, decorating the walls with pictures brought from home. But such kindnesses are incidental. They are kindnesses precisely because they are voluntary, something extra that individual members of the ICU staff may (or may
not) do, apart from the unit's primary task of treating acute physiological
disruptions. They are meant to get the patient—and, perhaps, the doctor or

nurse—through the day as comfortably as possible and with as little disruption of the real business of treatment as possible.

The Limits of Moral Judgment

In one curious sense, doctors and nurses do show an interest in their patients as persons. Despite their focus on physiology, the doctors and nurses who staff the intensive care units at Outerboro and Countryside do not shy away from moral judgment. When Tommy Jackson, a 26-year-old drug user on chronic dialysis, was admitted to the Outerboro unit, the unit physicians were quick to take me aside. "Here's a sociological problem," one told me. "It's not medical." And another explained, "He's been in the unit seven times and in the CCU three times. His basic stance is to whine. He's very dependent. . . . His mother is part of the problem. She thinks, my little Tommy. She doesn't believe he's ever done drugs." During the presentation of Jackson's case, the rest of the staff laughed when one of the interns reported that Jackson was claiming he no longer used drugs. And an attending physician, concerned about Jackson's hepatitis, suggested nothing less than that he should be given a visible stigmata of that high infectious disease: "I think they should be tattooed, frankly."

Tommy Jackson is an extreme case but by no means unique. The language of intensive care is filled with terms of derision. Perhaps the best known of these is GOME or GOMER, short for "get out of my Emergency Room," for a patient "who has lost—often through age—what goes into being a human being."[8] Even more starkly, I have heard comatose patients described as "dead meat" or "pets." Claims by drug users that they are no longer using drugs or by alcoholics that they are no longer drinking are dismissed routinely: "You never believe that," one resident announced during rounds. And one of the few times that I heard such a claim accepted, it was with high sarcasm: "I believe him. He's got no peripheral veins left." One demanding patient is described, with mock scientism, as "a roaring bear personality." Another patient, unemployed for five years and living in a men's shelter, is "absolutely pathetic." Yet others are "ornery," "crotchety," "crabby."

To be sure, the moral judgments cut both ways. Patients are characterized as "a nice lady," "a gentleman," "intelligent," "well educated," "a charmer,"

8. Samuel Shem, *The House of God* (New York: Dell, 1978), p. 424.

"patient," "a class act," "brave," and "cute." Occasionally, a resident will insist on the good standing of a patient: "He's a real citizen type. He works as a tailor. . . . He has a real job. He's not like Unknown Male." In one case, an intern was insistent even on distinguishing one drug user from the rest: "He was kind of a spiritual leader of the drug community."

Nonetheless, it is the negative characterizations which predominate. Like police officers preoccupied with crime or clergy preoccupied with sin, the physician's view draws disproportionately from the seamy side of life. Particularly in urban hospitals, and particularly in intensive care, a large proportion of the patients suffer from self-induced illness. Of the admissions I observed at Countryside, physicians included reports of drug use (9 percent), alcohol use (11 percent), or both (an additional 3 percent) in over one-fifth. Among 237 admissions at Countryside, the totals were even higher, with alcohol use reported in 18 percent of the cases, drug use in 8 percent, and both in an additional 3 percent. And none of this is to mention the suicide attempts, the frequent patient who had failed to follow a medically prescribed regimen, or the very frequent smoker. As medically relevant aspects of the patient's life, such behaviors are mentioned routinely in the initial presentation of the patient's social history. Although these presentations are usually quite matter of fact, their language insistently invokes the language of "abuse" and, by implication, evaluation: "social history notable for ethanol abuse," "a 53-year-old man with a history of alcohol abuse," "IV [intravenous] drug abuser with shortness of breath," "five-year history of IV drug abuse." Yet, even without the language of "abuse," the evaluative implications of such presentations are perhaps inevitable. Like the police and the clergy, physicians are not only licensed to view the seamy side of life but positively enjoined to seek it out. If, from this, there emerges a baleful, even cynical view of human life and human nature, it should not surprise us.

What might surprise us, however, is how little relevant the moral judgments of physicians and nurses are to life in intensive care. For the most part, the ICU staff neither demeans patients nor tries to reform them nor, most important, treats them differently on the basis of such judgments. Occasionally, a nurse or an intern may sit down with a patient and try to explain the health consequences of heavy drinking or drug use. So, too—and considerably less benignly—an occasional patient may be rushed out of the unit because the housestaff find him or her unusually distasteful. One patient, for example, according to an outraged Outerboro resident, had been sent out of the ICU "inappropriately" because, the resident thought, "she's an incredible pain in the ass . . . an alcoholic, active IV drug abuser, noncompliant with meds. . . . We don't like noncompliant people." But both differential treatment and efforts at reform are episodic and unsystematic. More frequent is a remarkably thoroughgoing tolerance, born perhaps of resignation. With all their complaints about Tommy Jackson, the ICU physicians nonetheless provided him with the hemodialysis he had come to the unit for and, finding his condition improved, at least temporarily, discharged him from the hospital. Doctors and nurses may make jokes among themselves about the wealthy patient whose cirrhosis of the liver was the result of too much Remy Martin Cognac or that one of the "drinking buddies" of a comatose woman was named "Jack Daniels." They may disbelieve the comatose man who, on awakening, insisted that he had never before used cocaine. But for the most part, they keep their jokes and disbeliefs to themselves. They address patients, except for the occasional ones who have lingered in the unit long enough to have assumed a first name, as "Mister" or "Mrs." or "Miss." Overwhelmed by acute medical crises, the ICU staff is simply too busy—and too little interested—to bother with reforming character. If they do not treat the liver disease that is a frequent source of gastrointestinal bleeding, they certainly do not even attempt to treat the alcoholism that is often the source of liver disease. If their job is to treat respiratory distress in a crisis situation, it matters little if the distress is the result of a cancer for which the patient is, to all appearances, blameless or the result of a drug-induced coma for which they would happily blame the patient.

Consider, for example, Naismith Brown. Brown is precisely the sort of patient who is frequently the butt of medical humor and the object of moral judgment. A 44-year-old single man with a long history of alcoholic cirrhosis, Brown was brought to Outerboro by the Emergency Medical Service with falling blood pressure, the result of a gastrointestinal bleed, itself brought on by too many drinks over too many years. In the Emergency Room, Brown was intubated for airway protection and sent almost immediately to the Intensive Care Unit. In the unit, Brown's doctors ordered an endoscopy, found the proximate source of his bleed, provided him with transfusions, prescribed pitressin to help control his bleeding, and, after a one-night stay, sent him to the wards for continued medical management.

Brown himself was alert and conscious throughout his ICU stay. But if anyone had spoken to him about his use of alcohol, if anyone had demeaned him, tried to reform him, or in any way distinguished him from the "solid citizens" who are the ICU staff's patients of preference, he could not remember:

Up there is strictly business place. What I mean by business place, you know, fast going place. But business place. So after they finish, after up there they finish the most important part of the job, they send you down, get your treatment. . . . They're very fast up there, and they know what they're doing. They know their work.

In Brown's vision of intensive care and in the vision of others like him, moral judgment has no part.

Moreover, it is a vision ICU physicians and nurses themselves whole-heartedly share. One addressed the situation of patients like Naismith Brown directly, comparing the practice of medicine in intensive care to that in other parts of the hospital:

We don't get very much involved with either their social problems or how they've responded to their disease or how they've gotten to the point that they're at. The classic is the alcoholic who's GI bleeding. We don't address the fact that, Is there anything that we can correct about their home situation or their social situation to stop them from drinking? Not that we could on the floor, but . . . that question isn't even addressed in the unit. What's addressed in the unit is how fast they're bleeding and where they're bleeding from.

Drugs and alcohol may bring patients to intensive care. And the physicians who treat those patients may disapprove, sometimes deeply, of the behaviors which are the underlying causes of the conditions they are called on to treat. But their job, at least as they see it, is not to reform behavior or even to distinguish among patients of widely varying character and imputed worth. The physicians in intensive care are not—and do not imagine themselves— as priests or cops, as ministers to the soul or guardians of decency. If anything, they are rather more like repairmen. If, in some circumstances, many of medicine's critics find such an image cold and impersonal, they must also recognize that it is, in other circumstances, egalitarian and even liberating.

The Patient Vanishes

In settings other than intensive care, what Anselm Strauss and his colleagues have called "sentimental work" assumes a prominent place in medical treatment. Successful treatment depends, integrally, on the physician's or nurse's ability to build trust, to help patients maintain their composure, to maintain or rebuild personal identities in the face of debilitating illness.[9] In such set-

9. Anselm Strauss, Shizuko Fagerhaugh, Barbara Suczek, and Carolyn Wiener, *The Social Organization of Medical Work* (Chicago: University of Chicago Press, 1985), especially pp. 129–50.

tings, a recognition of the patient's personhood is essential. But intensive care is different.

In intensive care, patients vanish. Patients do not, of course, vanish in the sense of disappearing physically. But they do vanish in two other senses. First, they vanish in the sense that disease itself robs them of many of the capabilities we associate with full personhood. Second, they vanish in the sense that the doctors and nurses who work in the unit are largely indifferent to matters of identity or character. "I have almost no relationship with the patients in the unit," an Outerboro resident explained. "If they're nice people, it's great. You kind of wave hello, whatever, but you don't have a whole lot of time . . . for small talk." This vanishing act is not a matter of design. Doctors and nurses do not start out with the intention of ignoring patients. Rather, other issues are simply more pressing.

The ICU staff live in a moral universe of limited liability. What happens before the patient enters intensive care may be of diagnostic interest, but it is not the housestaff's responsibility. What happens after the patient leaves the ICU may also be of interest, but neither is it part of the ICU's responsibility. Doctors and nurses attempt to restore their patients' personhood by medical treatment. But the restoration of personhood is, at best, an outcome of medical treatment. Personhood has little to do with the tasks at hand. Doctors and nurses—perhaps themselves overwhelmed by their patients' disease— do not imagine it as part of the process of treatment.

4

Doctors: The Banality of Heroism

Intensive care units are dense with doctors. At both Outerboro and Countryside there are unit attending physicians constantly in and out of the unit, always available by phone, "rounding" at Outerboro two or three hours every morning and, at Countryside, for an hour or so in the morning and again in the afternoon. There are private physicians following their own patients, albeit with varying degrees of energy and with varying degrees of deference to the unit attendings. There are consultants—cardiologists, pulmonologists, renal specialists, hematologists, neurologists—who come through the unit to share their special expertise. But most of all, there are the housestaff.[1]

At both Outerboro and Countryside, as at most teaching hospitals, housestaff provide twenty-four-hour coverage in intensive care. A Outerboro, the unit is staffed by three junior residents (two years past medical school) and four interns (one year past medical school). At Countryside, the medical service of the unit is staffed by a senior resident (three years out of medical school) and three interns in month-long rotations, with additional night coverage provided by senior residents drawn from other services. During the day, every day at Outerboro and every day but weekends at Countryside, the entire housestaff are present in the unit. At night, every night, one resident and two interns at Outerboro and one resident and one intern at Countryside are always available, physically present in the unit. The housestaff are the first people the nurses turn to when there is a sudden crisis, the first people consultants report their findings to, the first people private physicians check with. Other doctors come and go. The housestaff are always there.

The housestaff are central to the contemporary teaching hospital and,

1. It is not so everyplace. At many community hospitals without housestaff, private physicians assume responsibility for their own patients, visiting once in the morning and perhaps again in the afternoon. A staff physician, perhaps from the Emergency Room, may provide coverage in the event of a cardiac or respiratory arrest. Still, at many community hospitals, intensive care units are run, in effect, by nurses who provide the only continual coverage.

particularly, to intensive care. But the position of the housestaff is filled with ambiguities and tensions. As William Winkenwerder has observed, drawing on his own experience,

Residents are fully licenced to practice medicine, but they are not totally autonomous. They have heavy responsibilities in patients' care, but they are not independent in making many decisions. They are usually the primary caretakers, but usually not the ultimate decision makers.[2]

The housestaff are both practicing physicians and students. As practicing physicians, the housestaff are paid—decently by the standards of teachers or nurses but, with salaries ranging from twenty to thirty thousand dollars, poorly by the standards of more experienced physicians. At times, especially late at night, when no other physicians are around, and more so at Outerboro than at Countryside, the residents assume primary responsibility for patient care. At other times, these more often at Countryside than at Outerboro, the housestaff seem to be little more than overtrained messengers, assembling the judgments of consultants or the intentions of private physicians and then passing them along to the unit attendings. Still, especially for "service" patients (those without private physicians) but also for those patients whose private physicians do not actively manage cases in intensive care, the housestaff are, among the welter of consultants, the only "total patient persons."

But they are also students. It is, indeed, astonishing—not least, in retrospect, to the housestaff themselves—how little interns know, particularly at the beginning of the year. As one Outerboro resident recalled:

I had never seen a respirator in my life. You don't see any of that in medical school . . . unless you've done an ICU sub [a subinternship, a rotation during the fourth year of medical school], which I hadn't done. I remember I was terrified as a medical student. I said, "Oh, my God! If I don't do an ICU sub, what am I going to do when I go to an ICU?" Everybody tells you that it doesn't make any difference. They assume total ignorance. Which is true.

Teaching in the ICU, like clinical teaching in medicine more generally, is far from systematic. At Countryside there are special teaching rounds, which meet three times a week (following morning work rounds), and a "journal club," which meets once a week and at which the housestaff present reviews of recent articles. But the cases presented at teaching rounds and the articles reviewed in the journal club depend on who was admitted to the unit and with what problems. At Outerboro, teaching is even less systematic. There

2. William Winkenwerder, "Ethical Dilemmas for House Staff Physicians: The Care of Critically Ill and Dying Patients," *Journal of the American Medical Association* 254 (1985): 3454.

are no special teaching rounds, although a good deal of teaching is done during morning rounds. There is no journal club. At both Countryside and Outerboro, teaching is almost entirely case centered. Teaching consists of passing on the specific skills and knowledge—diagnostic, prognostic, therapeutic, and procedural—necessary to manage the particular patients in the unit at a particular time.

Despite its peculiarities, despite its hit or miss character, medical education, at least in the ICU, at least as a method of transmitting skills, seems to work. By the end of their training, the housestaff at both Outerboro and Countryside learn—among much else—how to set a ventilator, how to insert a Swan-Ganz catheter, how to interpret an electrocardiogram, how to manage pulmonary embolisms, acute renal failure, acute respiratory failure, sepsis, and shock.

It would be a mistake, however, to think of the education of housestaff as consisting solely of cognitive matters—of learning how to perform procedures or interpret data. It is also a moral education. On the face of it, this moral education is even less systematic than education about how to perform procedures, how to interpret data, or how to plan a course of action. Certainly, there is little formal training in ethics during internship or residency (or, for that matter, during medical school). Although more than a few discussions during teaching rounds do turn on questions of when it is right and proper to insist on informed consent, to discontinue treatment, to send one patient out of the unit rather than another, these discussions are even more situation specific than those concerning, for example, the management of patients on respirators or patients with severe kidney disease. Although, over the course of a year, an extraordinary range of ethically relevant issues is bound to come up in the management of actual cases, it is almost accidental whether a particular resident or intern will be rotating through the unit during the discussion of any particular issue.

The core of the housestaff's moral education is not in ethics so much as it is in values—not in learning how to reason like a philosopher or lawyer so much as in learning (and, perhaps, even internalizing) some of the basic assumptions, orientations, and concerns of physicians. Internship and residency (along with the final two, clinical years of medical school) occupy a special position in the moral imagination of physicians. Older physicians look back on their years as housestaff in the spirit of proud survivors and with the same strange mixture of reverence and disdain, nostalgia and revulsion that old soldiers reserve for basic training and combat. For those who go through them, internship and residency are extraordinarily intense experiences.

It is no doubt the intensity of the experience that explains the large number of firsthand accounts of clinical education in medicine. Like repentant sinners, doctors seem compelled to tell and retell the story of their third year of medical school, their internship, their residency, as if the act of confession will somehow purge themselves of their horror. Many of these accounts—most notably Konner's *Becoming a Doctor*, Harrison's *A Woman in Residence*, Shem's fictionalized *House of God*—are deeply critical of medical training.[3] But they are not critical of that training for its lack of moral education so much as for the negative character of that education—for teaching indifference to patients as well as for its constant onslaught on the identity of young physicians themselves. These are themes that have been picked up on by a number of somewhat more systematic sociological studies of medical training. Terry Mizrahi, in particular, has argued that the dominant perspective learned by housestaff, primarily from each other, consists of nothing less than an effort "to get rid of patients," both physically (by transferring them to another service or by assigning them to a hierarchical inferior) and mentally ("by objectifying, intimidating, or avoiding" them).[4]

Such claims that the primary moral lesson of clinical medical education is one of cynicism and indifference toward patients are too frequent and too insistent to be dismissed easily. Yet they are at best half-truths. While housestaff do learn cynicism and indifference, they learn other things as well. In particular, as Charles Bosk has emphasized in his superb study of surgical housestaff, a lack of "dedication, hard work, and proper reverence for role obligations"—all elements of "moral performance"—is judged more harshly than any failure of technical skill.[5] Above all, Bosk's housestaff learned "professional-self control," an "ability to handle responsibility" and an ability to restrain their own desires in favor of "the client's interest."[6]

The moral education of physicians is well-traveled terrain. But within this

3. Melvin Konner, *Becoming a Doctor* (New York: Viking, 1987); Michelle Harrison, *A Woman in Residence* (New York: Random House, 1982); Samuel Shem, *The House of God* (New York: Dell, 1978). For a review of this literature, see Peter Conrad, "Learning to Doctor: Reflections on Recent Accounts of the Medical School Years," *Journal of Health and Social Behavior* 29 (1988): 323–32.

4. Terry Mizrahi, *Getting Rid of Patients* (New Brunswick, NJ: Rutgers University Press, 1986), p. 167. Also see her "Coping with Patients: Subcultural Adjustments to the Conditions of Work among Internists-in-Training," *Social Problems* 1984 (32): 156–66, and Diana Scully, *Men Who Control Women's Health: The Miseducation of Obstetricians and Gynecologists* (Boston: Houghton Mifflin, 1980).

5. Charles Bosk, *Forgive and Remember: Managing Medical Failure* (Chicago: University of Chicago Press, 1979), p. 175.

6. Ibid., p. 182.

terrain, intensive care occupies a particularly strategic vantage point. It is in intensive care that the stresses and strains of housestaff training, that the temptation to look indifferently on patients, and that the opportunity to develop collective coping mechanisms all reach their high point. The rotation through intensive care is that moment in clinical training at which housestaff are both most susceptible to a moral education and most in need of it.

The End of Idealism

Doctors, like the practitioners of any occupation, enter medicine for a wide range of motives and reasons. However, unlike most occupations, unlike even most other professional occupations, medicine requires an unusually early commitment. Because of the demands of premedical programs, along with the long haul of medical school and residency, future doctors typically begin their training early, at the beginning of college, at the age of 17 or 18. Moreover, because of its prestige and generous compensation, medicine is a favorite occupation of parents ambitious for their children. As a result, many doctors, including many of the interns and residents at both Outerboro and Countryside, are only dimly aware of when, let alone why, they decided to go into medicine. As one usually articulate Outerboro resident, momentarily unable to formulate thoughts with his typical precision, told me, "I had for a long time, growing up, this feeling that I was going to be a doctor." He could specify his career choice no further.

Although many of the interns and residents are unaware of why they went into medicine, they nonetheless entered with expectations. Certainly, most expected to be paid well and to be respected for their efforts. But some expected something more as well. Medicine seemed to represent an almost unique opportunity to combine high intellectual, particularly scientific, activity with service to humankind. As one resident told me, "One of the reasons I went into medicine was because it had to do with trying to bring together social issues with other issues." And as another, Lynn, added, "I thought it was the ideal combination of work where I could help people, interact with people, both patients and lots of colleagues, and do science, which I love."

Yet those who entered medicine in the spirit of lofty ideals quickly found their expectations disappointed.[7] Lynn, for example, had found that medi-

7. The "end of idealism" theme is an old one in studies of medical students and housestaff. The classic statement is Howard S. Becker and Blanche Geer, "The Fate of Idealism in Medical School," *American Sociological Review* 23 (1958): 50–56. See also Howard Becker, Blanche Geer,

cine did meet some of her expectations: "It certainly is a job with a lot of intellectual sides to it. You do deal with a lot of people." But while Lynn had by no means abandoned her original idealism, she was no longer so sure that medicine was the right place to express it. In the first place, she had been surprised by how demanding her residency and internship had been:

I think what I didn't anticipate was the depth of responsibility that you really do have for other people's lives and how much I really did or didn't want that. . . . I also didn't anticipate the work load, which I don't think anybody did. In fact, that's the major difference between what you fantasize and what actually happens.

But even more, she had been surprised by the transformation in her attitude toward the very patients she had gone into medicine to help.

Then there's all the social problems. I was very idealistic, and I felt I had an obligation to the poor. And even if I didn't envision myself working in a clinic in a poor area completely, I always felt that I would do a certain amount of that to balance out what has been given to me. I didn't anticipate how much the social problems of the patients here would make other kinds of caring difficult and how just being overwhelmed by the system, the bureaucracy, and the social problems of these patients would kind of make you feel dragged down and, to a certain extent, lose interest.

Lynn was certainly unusual in the extent of her original idealism. Yet her frustrations and declining interest in many of the patients she was called on to help were echoed widely by interns and residents at both Outerboro and Countryside. Nowhere are these frustrations more acute than in intensive care.

Everyone Your Enemy

For a house officer in intensive care, the most fundamental fact of life is fatigue. At Countryside, which enjoys a reputation for sponsoring unusually "humane" internships and residencies, rotations through the Intensive Care Unit last for one month and are repeated twice in the course of the year. During their month in the unit, interns and residents report for work every morning well before nine o'clock and remain in the unit until late afternoon or early evening. In addition, both interns and residents are "on call" every third day and stay in the unit the entire evening and night. Only on Saturdays and Sundays, and then only on those weekend days when they are not either coming off an on-call night or preparing for one (which is to say one day out

---

Everett Hughes, and Anselm Strauss, *Boys in White: Student Culture in Medical School* (Chicago: University of Chicago Press, 1961).

of three), can the Countryside house officers avoid the hospital altogether. In an average week, an intern or resident will spend roughly eighty-five hours in the unit and in a typical month will be in the unit for at least part of the day for twenty-eight of thirty-one days.

At Outerboro, the unit rotation is only two weeks long, but is repeated three times over the course of the year and is even more rigorous than at Countryside. As at Outerboro, the residents are on call every third night. The day after their on-call night, they can leave the unit immediately after morning rounds, usually sometime between eleven o'clock and noon. The day before, they are on "short call" and are expected to stay in the unit until early evening. The interns are on call every other night and are expected to stay in the unit even on the days after their on-call nights until they have finished writing their notes, usually sometime in early to mid-afternoon. Weekends are no different from weekdays, and, except to accompany patients to procedures performed outside the unit ("field trips"), neither residents nor interns are supposed to leave the unit at any time while they are on call. Even their meals are brought in on trays. Over the course of a week, then, both residents and interns at Outerboro will spend nearly one hundred hours in the unit and will be in the unit at least part of the day every day for two weeks.

At both Countryside and Outerboro, special on-call rooms—one for each intern and resident at Countryside, a single room for all three house officers at Outerboro—provide the housestaff at least the opportunity to sleep, even during on-call nights. But these Spartan rooms are used lightly. "You know, you try to sleep at night," one resident reflected after his last rotation through the unit. But "it wasn't a good sleep. You were always waking up at regular intervals and worrying about something." Residents and interns alike probably average between two and four hours of sleep a night when they are on call. Some nights they get more. Many nights they sleep not at all.[8]

8. The effects of housestaff rotations are not limited to fatigue. Although rotations are often justified by "continuity of care," the irony is that they create considerable discontinuity. Especially at Outerboro—with its two-week rotations accompanied by alternating days on and off—interns and residents alike are constantly "picking up" patients they have not themselves admitted. And because, as one resident told me, "you know the patients you admitted personally a lot better," the collective memory of the Outerboro unit may occasionally fail in matters that are not raised repeatedly on rounds or reiterated in chart notes. Although the admitting intern may have been careful to explain that a patient was a drug user or an altogether solid citizen, such information may easily be forgotten by successive teams of interns and residents more concerned with managing acute physiological problems than the conditions that brought the patient to the unit in the first place. Thus, the daily rotations at both Outerboro and Countryside and the biweekly or monthly rotations, particularly at Outerboro, discourage physicians from concen-

To the lack of sleep is added the burden of responsibility, particularly for the residents. "As an intern last year," one resident explained,

it was a very structured environment, very protected. There were always people there to ask questions. . . . Then I became a resident and the responsibilities change a little bit. I've only done the medical unit once so far, and there's a lot more responsibility. You're sort of on the other side of the fence, where you have two new interns who are always asking you questions. The stress is a little greater. At nighttime you feel a little bit more alone in that you're the one that has to make the decision.

Another resident, Stuart, compared the unit to other rotations:

There's a lot more pressure as a resident in the ICU than on the wards or anyplace else. The only other place where there's a lot of pressure is the Emergency Room, but as a junior resident, it's not as bad as when you're in ICU. I think the reason is you really have to decide, you're always getting bothered, sort of badgered by everyone as the person in charge. . . . You're responsible for everything that goes on.

Or, as yet another resident put it, "It can be scary."

If the constant lack of sleep might be bearable but for the responsibilities of the unit rotation, so, too, might the responsibilities be bearable but for the constant frustrations of intensive care medicine. Although roughly two-thirds of admissions leave the hospital alive at both Outerboro and Countryside, those who die without leaving the hospital are characterized by longer ICU stays. As a result, despite the housestaff's best efforts, roughly every other bed at Outerboro and Countryside is filled with a patient who will eventually die without leaving the hospital.

"Because," one resident explained, "there are so very few who make it through," the satisfactions of the unit come "more from your peers than from your patients." "Mostly," she continued, "all you see is a lot of death. And death is not gratifying." Even the patients who do survive provide only slightly more satisfaction. "You have to get self-gratification," another resident suggested. "You don't get it from the patients because they are so sick that they don't know what they've come through. They don't know how sick they've been." As one resident summed up his experience:

It's a very stressful place to work. The people there are very sick and you are responsible for them and a lot of things can happen. You are just very, you're very hyper a lot of the times and you feel very, very pressured for most of the time you're there. . . . It's also the amount of work you put into it. . . . It's not as satisfying, simply because

---

trating on long-term goals: "Because of the way we rotate through the unit and the scheduling we do, we're happy [if] the person lives through another day." In this sense, the pattern of rotations contributes to the focus on acute physiological problems that I argued, in the previous chapter, is characteristic of intensive care medicine more generally.

there's a lack of personal interaction with the patients. . . . Sometimes you walk through there and you feel like you're part of a large science experiment on humans because all these things are going on. . . . So it's a very hard place to work for the reason that it's so stressful and so relatively unsatisfying.

Despite everything, some interns and residents do occasionally become deeply attached to particular patients. Larry, one of the Countryside interns, told me that he had identified strongly with one of his patients, a woman of roughly his own age who had been admitted to the unit early in his rotation. But Larry did not see his emotional involvement in the case as a virtue. Quite the reverse. He told me, "If you are involved with the patient, you're going to become emotionally drained and burned out very soon. . . . As a physician, as a nurse, as a health care professional, you can't be emotionally involved with your patients. . . . If you are not objective about your patients, you can't take care of them."

The dangers Larry raised—one response to the dilemmas of what Renee Fox has called, more generally, detached concern—are, of course, endemic to young physicians everywhere.[9] But they are particularly acute in the ICU because of the high death rate among unit patients and the intensity of treatment. Thus, housestaff pull away from potential relationships with patients in intensive care not only because they care too little but also because of the dangers of caring too much. "Usually," an Outerboro resident told me, "you can't talk to them. Usually, and there's no question about this, if you can talk to them, you wish you couldn't, not because you're busy as much as the fact that you're torturing them."

Given the stress of internships and residencies in medicine, and the ICU in particular, it is hardly surprising that some house officers try to withdraw from their responsibilities. Although the dropout rate from internships and residencies is remarkably low (most likely a consequence of the long commitment to pre-med training and medical school that precedes the internship), one Outerboro intern did, in fact, come close to dropping out of the program altogether during his ICU rotation and was able to finish only one of his scheduled two weeks in the unit. More often, though, houses officers withdraw psychologically rather than administratively. As Stuart explained,

9. Renee C. Fox and Harold I. Leif, "Training for Detached Concern in Medical Students," pp. 12–35, in Harold Lief, Victor F. Lief, and Nina R. Lief, *The Psychological Basis of Medical Practice* (New York: Harper & Row, 1963). For a discussion of detached concern in intensive care, see Robert H. Coombs and Lawrence Goldman, "Maintenance and Discontinuity of Coping Mechanisms in an Intensive Care Unit," *Social Problems* 20 (1973): 342–55.

Initially, I think, in the beginning of this junior year it was somewhat exciting and you kind of, you were in charge and if everyone lived you felt pretty good, or if you did things well you felt pretty good. At this point I'm starting to get just a little bit more uninterested in that and more interested in being able to be awake when I get home or be able to relate to my wife or something.

Neither is it surprising, given all this, that the housestaff often lose sympathy for the very patients they are, ostensibly, in the unit to help. "Last year," one resident told me,

in the other unit [the Cardiac Care Unit] the juniors were there for a month straight and they were going bonkers. They were on [call] every other [day]; they weren't on every third. At the end of the four months they were going bonkers. People whom I liked would say things like, "This patient shouldn't be in the unit because he only speaks Spanish." They would just get completely inappropriate and burned out and hostile.

As one intern told me, "The first thing you learn is that everyone is your enemy." The products of fatigue and frustration, then, are withdrawal, anger toward patients, and cynicism.

Puzzles, Games, and Responsibility

The withdrawal from responsibility, the anger toward patients, and the cynicism are all too significant and too much a part of the housestaff's experience to ignore. But they are only part of the story. What is perhaps more surprising than the housestaff's fatigue and frustration is their general eagerness— albeit to greater or lesser degree and with occasional exceptions—to meet the responsibilities that are thrust upon them even in remarkably trying circumstances.

The importance of meeting those responsibilities is taught in part, and as Bosk found among the surgical housestaff he studied, by attendings.

Mr. Delgado, an 80-year-old man admitted to the Outerboro unit with Hodgkin's disease and renal disease, had gone to emergency surgery late at night for a gastro-intestinal bleed. The next morning, Jimmy, the resident who had been on at night, explained that Delgado's private physician had made the decision. Dennis, the unit director, was unhappy. "I don't know how these things get started, and this year there have been a lot, but this has got to stop. It must make sense to you that Jimmy, who's been seeing this patient, makes the decision." The private [physician], he continued, "hasn't seen the patient for a week. We can't ask them to make every critical decision when they aren't here." Private physicians, Dennis recognized, might put pressure on residents to go along with them. But even this, he insisted, was no reason to back off.

As long as the residents assumed responsibility, he would support them. "Don't make it a turf battle. It's his [Delgado's] problem. If you think you know what's best for the patient, say your attending will call. . . . Look, every other night is still burned into my brain, even in my dotage. A full night's sleep is still a blessing. Better you call me at night than that I find out about it in the morning."

Ken, the medical director of the Countryside unit, had been glancing at the chart of Mrs. Schmidt, a 67-year-old woman with chronic pulmonary disease and a long history of heart attacks. When he noticed that there had not been an X-ray taken after the placement of a Swan-Ganz catheter, he exploded. "It's uncalled for. I'm asking for minimal things." He glared at the interns. "When you are residents next year, you'd goddamned better be demanding of your interns. . . . You should not have to be pushed at this time in your career. There's no reason that basic things cannot be done." He glared at the resident. "You have to as a resident take hold of things and say this is how things have to be done. . . . I don't get upset when they infarcted their lungs by mistake. That's just part of the system. But I do get upset when minimal things don't get done."

Attendings do not expect the housestaff to be right all the time. They do not expect them to understand everything about intensive care medicine. But they do expect the housestaff to acknowledge their limits and ask for help when they need it. "If you don't know what's going on," Ken insisted, "you should call the intensivist on call. Those of you who get lousy evaluations are the ones who don't call, no matter how smart you are." And, most of all, they expect the housestaff to assume responsibility. "The truth is," one Outerboro attending insisted when a resident suggested that a nurse had made a near fatal mistake, "the doctor has the responsibility." Ken echoed this sentiment at Countryside: "You should start taking control of your own patients." The housestaff accept responsibility, in part, because their attendings insist that they do.

But even more important than the insistences of attendings are the lessons that interns and residents teach each other. At both Outerboro and Countryside, the intensive care rotation stands out as the single moment in the entire training program during which relations among housestaff are most intense. Outside the hospital, there is considerable variation in how friendly the housestaff are with each other—ranging from a few couples who are either married or living together to others who rarely see any colleagues in social situations. On other rotations, particularly on the wards, interns and residents work, for the most part, independently, particularly of other housestaff of their own year. Inside the unit, however, they are almost all, if not friends, at least comrades:

One of the best parts of this program is the camaraderie we have. I feel very close to many of the seniors and many of the interns. . . . It's a closer relationship because in most other rotations as the junior resident, at least, you're on your own. It's you supervising the interns. . . . The units are sort of unique in that you're there with another one of your equals.

The best thing about this residency program is the other people. It's really the only good thing about this residency program. It's one of the major reasons I've always loved working in the unit. It's fun to work with the other housestaff, the interns and the residents.

The housestaff are thrown together physically in the unit, eating together, sleeping side by side, with a degree of intimacy usually reserved for lovers. As one resident put it, "It's kind of like you're . . . roughing it together." But even more important, the housestaff depend on each other. "The two of you," one Outerboro resident observed of the long-call/short-call system,

aren't there all night because someone goes home at eight. But you don't make any major interventions or major decisions without your colleague being there. That, most of the time, the great majority of the time, it's a comfort. I think you derive strength from each other by being there.

When the housestaff do not work well together, an already difficult rotation becomes even more so. "I can think of one particular rotation," one Outerboro resident remembered.

The problem was the other, the resident was my short resident. I was long on the day that he would cover short. Instead of working as a team, I felt like he was working as a rival almost and would look up labs and then not tell me about them. Instead of my idea of what a short resident is there for . . . , to make the life of a long resident as easy as possible and prepare that person for the night when they're alone. But it's very much a team effort. You share whatever information you get, especially since that person . . . should know as much as possible. So the combination of that, collecting that kind of information and not letting me know, and also just, I remember making recommendations and literally being basically laughed at. It was a personality problem. . . . It's just totally unproductive, and it's not fun.

Such conflicts are perhaps inevitable among any group of people as aggressive and strong-willed as the Outerboro and Countryside housestaff. But fortunately they are, by most accounts, rare. "Most of the people in our program," an resident pointed out, "really go out of their way to be considerate to their fellow housestaff. I think there's a sense of camaraderie that's generated in the unit because it is a very difficult rotation."

Given the heavy burden of work that falls on them collectively, the housestaff are particularly intent on sharing that burden equitably and fairly. Thus, at both Outerboro and Countryside, interns usually accept new patients in strict turns. However, in both units, when, by chance, one intern accumulates significantly more than his or her share of the unit's patients (a matter of having accepted one or two patients whose unit stay is significantly longer than average), the resident will typically reassign one or more patients to equalize the burden. If interns or residents know in advance that they will miss a day for some special reason, they usually make arrangements to trade a night on call with another house officer. Even more important, interns and residents alike reserve a special scorn for those of their colleagues they feel are shirking.

Charles had called in sick at Countryside. A day and a half before, he had had a temperature of 102 but had stayed on call all night. When I told him—sympathetically but perhaps without a good deal of understanding—that he should go home, he said he'd missed some days earlier in the year and didn't want to miss any more. The morning that Charles called in sick, Dave, the unit resident, Larry, one of the other interns, and Peter, a resident who had stopped by to say hello to Dave, were making jokes about this having happened before. Larry, who seemed particularly angry, told me that he didn't doubt that Charles was sick, but somebody else has to work for him and that's not fair. He, Larry, had worked one day when he was vomiting. He went down to the Emergency Room, got a shot to stop vomiting, and slept for two hours but kept on working. Dave told me that he, himself, had missed only two days in three years. The next day Charles was still out sick, and at the beginning of rounds Ken asked where he was. Dave explained that Charles was still sick. But Ken was hardly sympathetic. "Still? Friday, Saturday, Sunday. No one is sick for three, four days. I won't stand for that." But hearing criticism from an attending, Dave closed ranks, adding that Charles had a fever and sore throat and had been to the Emergency Room.

The incident is a telling one. Dave, Peter, and particularly Larry (who stood to suffer most from Charles's absence) were scornful of Charles for shirking despite an excuse (his illness) that would, in almost any other circumstance, be considered entirely legitimate. However, when Ken criticized Charles, Dave defended him, suggesting, implicitly, that it was a concern for the housestaff themselves. Moreover, Charles himself had anticipated the reaction his absence would provoke. (When he came back to work on Monday, he asked me if anyone had said anything.) There is, then, a clear consensus. Any shirking of responsibilities, even the hint of shirking, may be defended against attendings but will be severely censured by the other housestaff themselves.

There is a threat implicit in the consensus. If an intern shirks responsibility, the resident and the other interns will not help him when he needs help. If a resident shirks responsibility, the other residents (at Outerboro) will not help her nor (at either Outerboro or Countryside) will her interns make the extra effort they might make for another resident. Indeed, for the occasional intern or, even more rarely, resident who does not meet his or her responsibilities, the ICU rotation becomes a special and lonely misery. Thus, the housestaff not only teach responsibility. They enforce it.

It is important, however, to recognize the character of this responsibility. It is not responsibility of the sort stressed by attendings, based on abstract obligations to patients. Rather, it is responsibility to other housestaff, based on very concrete relationships and mutual dependence. But it is the peculiar genius of medical training that the implications of these two very different types of responsibility for behavior are often very much the same. Moreover, the acceptance of responsibility is only one of several instances in which the very mechanisms housestaff develop to cope with the demands of their training are turned to the service of patients.

Sociologists have been quick to point to situations in which the internal interests of occupations and organizations have undermined their expressed purposes—how mental hospitals, for example, sacrifice patient care to the convenience of staff or how the military may sacrifice national security to the exigencies of officers' careers. We have been perhaps somewhat less likely to recognize the ways in which the interests of occupations and organizations, and of the people who staff them, may actually contribute to their purposes, even in slightly altered form. In the case of medicine, some observers have argued that physicians' loyalty to each other may interfere with the provision of effective patient care. While this undoubtedly is the case in some instances, I have suggested that, at least in intensive care, responsibility to other house officers is the means by which responsibility to patients is enforced. Some observers have argued that medical students, interns, and residents alike often pursue their own education to the detriment of patients whose cases are "not interesting." In contrast, I would suggest—again, at least in intensive care—that an emphasis on training opportunities is the means by which housestaff motivate themselves to provide care under what would otherwise be nearly intolerable stress.

Indeed, despite the stresses, many of the interns and residents at both Outerboro and Countryside actually prefer intensive care to their other rotations. Although there are other reasons for this preference (including, for some, the very lack of patient contact), the most important is that the unit offers unique opportunities to learn. "It's the only place in the hospital where you can put a Swan line in and an A line in [catheters used to monitor heart functions]," one resident explained. "I like that portion of it." On the "floor," the medical wards that are the location for long stretches of internship and residency at both Outerboro and Countryside, many of the patients have what the housestaff quickly come to think of as routine problems. In contrast, the unit often has "very interesting cases." Moreover, the intense monitoring that is a hallmark of intensive care provides the housestaff with a kind and quantity of data that is not otherwise available. "I liked the idea," another resident explained,

that you had real control over the patient, in the sense that you control their respiration, their blood pressure, their heart rates sometimes, and you had information on the pressures in the lungs and everything else and that you really weren't treating a patient in an unscientific way, which I thought was very fascinating and exciting.

To many of the housestaff, fascinated to begin with by the scientific analysis of disease, the intensive care unit offers precisely what they had been looking for in medicine. "In the unit," according to one resident, "with somebody with congestive heart failure, you put in the Swan and you're following the wedge [a measure of heart function]. On the floor you might use some medicines and listen to their lungs and wait a couple of days and then change the medicines." Questions, she continued, of, for example, why

the blood pressure [is] low really make you think about physiology as you were taught in medical school, which I never understood in medical school. I mean, it was a wonderful feeling to finally understand Swans. When you put in a Swan, it's like the problems that you got in medical school. It's like you're watching physiology.

In contrast, "On the floor you're kind of waiting for the patient to get better a little bit more." Another added that he had "learned as much in the ICU . . . in the six weeks I was there as I did on the floors." Thus, the stress of patient care in the unit is justified, by the housestaff themselves, by its contribution to their training.

This is not simply a matter of justifying present discomforts for future gains. It is also a matter of enjoying intensive care itself. The very complexity of caring for acutely ill patients takes on something of the character of a game. And in much the same spirit as they would approach a crossword or jigsaw puzzle, many of the interns and residents come to treat patient care much as they would approach a game. Caring for acutely ill patients, even under conditions of fatigue, even with the knowledge that they are likely to die, can actually become enjoyable. A unit patient may become, as one resident told me, "an object on the bed with lots of tubes and monitors and blood pressure." Moreover, he added, particularly as a resident, "you hardly examine them except for the data they come in with. So it becomes very much an intellectual problem." But even without any knowledge of or concern for the patient as a person, the game-like quality of intensive care sustains interest in the case: "They have interesting problems. The multisystem. It's kind of a puzzle. It's fun." Another resident made similar observations:

> You use your formulas, and then you kind of know what medicines to use. And you watch the numbers change as you use them, the way they're supposed to. Of course, they don't always work the way they're supposed to. It's fun in the way a science project is fun. It's fun the way, if you enjoy doing math problems in school, it's very much the same.

The game-like quality of intensive care medicine allows the residents to maintain their efforts on behalf of patients they might otherwise have little interest in. It also allows them to maintain their efforts in the face of the frustrations of frequent death. "I view it as a game . . . when . . . I disagree with them being up here and the only way that I can do it emotionally is to say that this is not a person. It's a piece of meat. It's a physiology experiment and let's do it!" Moreover, like any game, the game of patient care may take on competitive aspects. In discussing why continued efforts are made on be-half of moribund patients, one resident suggested

> that it's a selfish reason. You know, you try to keep them alive because you're the one that saved this person. I don't know how much it was done because they actually thought they could bring this person back to [being] a viable human being more than we got him to live during his stay in the ICU. In a competitive place where these people pride themselves on being such good doctors, that idea is sometimes prevalent.

If, more generally, the housestaff are frustrated by their inability to do more for dying patients, games provide their own justification. As Michael Burawoy has pointed out in a different context, "The very activity of playing a game generates consent with respect to its rules. . . . The game becomes an end in itself, overshadowing, masking, and even inverting the conditions out of which it emerged." [10] In the context of intensive care, a game-like ori-entation is produced by indifference. Only because the housestaff do not know or think of their patients as full people can they think of the medical care they provide as a "physiology experiment." Yet, at the same time, think-ing of care as a game, a puzzle, or an experiment allows the housestaff to maintain a level of energy that operates in the interest of the patient.

10. Michael Burawoy, *Manufacturing Consent* (Chicago: University of Chicago Press, 1979), p. 82.

The Banality of Heroism

On July 1, 1989, new regulations went into effect in New York state, limiting housestaff to shifts no longer than twenty-four hours and to a maximum of eighty hours of work a week.[11] A response to a few prominent cases in which exhausted, unsupervised house officers appeared to provide blatantly dangerous care, the regulations were intended to eliminate some of the worst abuses of medical training. As I write, it is too early to know whether the New York regulations—likely to be adopted in other states as well—will have their intended effect. (My own, unsubstantiated expectation is that they will ultimately benefit both patients and physicians.) What is clear, however, is that, whatever the eventual balance of benefits and costs, something will have been lost.

The fatigue and anxiety of housestaff training are fundamental to the moral education of physicians. This moral education does not consist of abstract principles. Neither does it consist of lessons taught by more senior physicians. Rather, in the very course of adapting to the stresses of their training, housestaff learn from each other. Moreover, what the housestaff learn are standards distinct not only to physicians but to physicians at a particular stage of their careers. They learn to value not responsibility to patients but responsibility to each other. They learn to value medical care not for its benefits to patients but for its training opportunities and as an encapsulated intellectual challenge. These are not the values likely to be of foremost concern to the patients who arrive at hospitals seeking medical attention. They are instead values of primary importance to the occupation of medicine, values that generate and maintain commitment to that occupation regardless of its explicit claims to patient service. In some instances, the housestaff's emphasis on responsibility to each other and on training opportunities (along with the hospital's reliance on housestaff as a relatively inexpensive source of skilled labor) may conflict with responsibility to patients or effective patient care. More often, however, at least in intensive care, responsibility of the housestaff to each other is the mode by which responsibility to patients is enforced and an emphasis on training or the game-like quality of medicine provides the motivation to maintain high levels of effort in the face of frequent frustrations.

The housestaff are heroic. Exhausted and frightened, they nonetheless

11. For a discussion of the New York regulations and some of their implications, see Kenneth E. Thorpe, "House Staff Supervision and Working Hours," *Journal of the American Medical Association* 263 (1990): 3177–81.

appear in the unit every morning, wake up in the middle of the night to pound on the chest of a patient whose heart has ceased to beat on its own, and run tests and procedures, compulsively, even on patients with only the slimmest chance of survival. But there is also, to borrow a phrase, a banality to their heroism. The housestaff are not heroic through any special strength of character. There is no reason to think that the housestaff at Outerboro and Countryside are significantly more (or less) virtuous than any other more or less random assortment of men and women in their mid-twenties. Rather, they are heroic because medical training and the hospital require them to be so. If they are heroic, they are heroic in the routine course of doing their jobs, preparing for the future, and getting through the day. It is the genius of medical training that it turns such banal concerns to such lofty ends.

5

The Nurse's Dilemma

Who would have believed . . . that the nurses were so much more important to sick people than the doctors were? Doctors didn't know that at all. As a doctor, he had always thought of the nurse—it astonished him now that he could have been so dense—as a sort of executive secretary. If she (always she) kept an orderly desk, knew what was going on with the patients, took orders efficiently and gave the right pill to the right patient at the right time, she was a good nurse.

But now that he was a patient, he could see that the nurses were . . . angels! Angels of mercy!

They were with him constantly, these women figures. They were gentle and good. They fixed his pillow. They came when he called for help. They said "This will make you feel better" and "There, isn't that better?" They touched him with their hands, flesh to flesh. His succor. His lifesavers. His lifelines.

Martha Lear, Heartsounds[1]

Perhaps.

In recent years, a number of sociologists and historians have grown rather insistent that their colleagues interested in health, medicine, and illness have given short shrift to nurses. They point out, quite rightly, that, while there are many fine studies of physicians, both historical and contemporary, there are few of nurses.[2]

1. Martha Lear, *Heartsounds* (New York: Simon & Schuster, 1980), pp. 38, 39.
2. The handful includes, among historical studies, Barbara Melosh, *The Physician's Hand* (Philadelphia: Temple University Press, 1982); Susan Reverby, *Ordered to Care: The Dilemma of American Nursing, 1850–1945* (Cambridge: Cambridge University Press, 1987); David Wagner, "The Proletarianization of Nursing in the United States, 1932–1946," *International Journal of Health Services* 10 (1980): 271–90; Ellen Condliffe Lagemann, ed., *History of Nursing: New Perspectives, New Directions* (New York: Teachers College Press, 1978). Among studies of contemporary nurses, see Zane Robinson Wolf, *Nurses' Work, the Sacred and the Profane* (Philadelphia: University of Pennsylvania Press, 1988), and Peggy Anderson, *Nurse* (New York: Berkley Books, 1978).

The recent interest in nurses, albeit still little more than a trickle, is not hard to explain. First, nurses significantly outnumber physicians and the growth rate of nursing is significantly faster. As late as the 1920s, there were as many physicians practicing in the United States as there were nurses. But by 1980, nurses outnumbered physicians by a ratio of three to one, with over one million registered nurses in the United States as well as an additional half million licensed practical nurses, compared to under a half million physicians. Second, interest in nursing is an expression of a more general interest in the participation of women in the labor force. Nursing is, and always has been, a woman's occupation. Although a very few more men are entering nursing than was the case as recently as 1980, their numbers remain small. At the end of the 1980s, 97 percent of registered nurses were women.[3] Thus, nursing has become an important case in the study of the gender-based division of labor. Third, the interest in nurses reflects a more general renewal of interest in the dynamics of the labor process in large-scale organizations. Technically skilled, but employed predominantly within and dependent on the large hospital, nurses (along with engineers, accountants, and craft workers) have become a critical case in the study of rationalization and deskilling at the workplace.

All of these are compelling reasons for studying nurses. None, however, are even weak reasons for making nurses central to the study of health care. Numbers alone do not make an occupation important, if those numbers are not converted to influence. So, too, while the female composition of nursing makes it important to the study of the gender-based division of labor and the organizational employment of nursing makes it important to the study of occupations and professions, neither characteristic necessarily makes nursing important to the study of health care unless those characteristics are the source of a distinctive voice.

The claim that nursing has been insufficiently studied, at least from the point of view of those interested in health care, rests on rather narrower grounds: that nurses, because they are women, because of their position in the organization of the hospital, do represent a distinctive voice, one otherwise little heard in contemporary American medicine. It is this claim that is put forward by Martha Lear in the plaintive account of her physician husband's illness cited at the beginning of this chapter. It is a claim put perhaps most explicitly by Renee Fox:

3. American Nurses Association, *Facts about Nursing, 1986–87* (New York: American Nurses Association, 1987).

In their daily, hands-on, continuous care of patients, nurses deal with some of their most basic and intimate physical, emotional, and, not infrequently, spiritual needs. They come to know patients in these outer and inner ways—especially how patients are reacting to and dealing with their illness and treatment. Nurses also have considerable contact with close members of patients' families. Under these circumstances, they often become identified with their patients as persons: with their feelings, values, relationships, life histories, and how these bear on what the hospitalized patient is experiencing. In fact, the nurse is ideally expected to do so, and to translate this identification into patient advocacy when it is called for.[4]

To some, the special role of the nurse emanates from the putatively distinctive female virtues of sympathy and nurturance. To others, it depends on an organizational mandate. But whatever its sources, Fox and others envision a distinctive role for nurses—"angels of mercy," more concerned with the social and emotional aspects of illness than are their more narrowly technical counterparts, the physicians, and effective advocates for more humane treatment.

All this is well and good. Unfortunately, it bears little resemblance to the role of nurses in the intensive care units at Outerboro and Countryside hospitals.

Nursing and Intensive Care

In some senses, the intensive care units at Outerboro and Countryside, like intensive care units more generally, may be understood as nursing units. Intensive care, as I suggested in chapter 2, began as an organizational innovation intended to concentrate nursing care on critically ill patients. On most shifts, at both Outerboro and Countryside, there is more than one nurse for every two patients. On average, intensive care units employ three times as many nurses per patient as do general medical and surgical wards.[5]

Moreover, it is nurses who provide the greatest part of whatever stability is to be found among intensive care personnel. At Outerboro, attending physicians rotate through the unit for a month at a time. At both Outerboro and

4. Fox, *Sociology of Medicine*, p. 60. Variants on this claim can be found in Renee C. Fox, Linda H. Aiken, and Carla M. Messikomer, "The Culture of Caring: AIDS and the Nursing Profession," *Milbank Quarterly* 68 (1990): 226–56; Melosh, *Physician's Hand;* Reverby, *Ordered;* Anderson, *Nurse;* and, in a rigorous study of nurses and physicians in a neonatal intensive care unit, Renee Anspach, "Prognostic Conflict in Life-and-Death Decisions: The Organization as an Ecology of Knowledge," *Journal of Health and Social Behavior* 28 (1987): 215–31.

5. Louise Russell, *Technology in Hospitals: Medical Advances and Their Diffusion* (Washington, DC: Brookings Institution, 1979), p. 46.

Countryside, new cohorts of interns and residents appear in the unit every year and stay for rotations of only two weeks or a month. In contrast, the nurses are in the unit three days a week, twelve hours a day, often for years at a stretch. Even on the Outerboro day shift, which has a reputation among the nurses there as a high turnover shift, several nurses had been working in the unit for nearly a decade; one of the night shift nurses had been working in the unit for fourteen years and several others for more than a decade. At Countryside, three nurses had each been working in the unit for over fifteen years. Although the continued expansion of both units generates a constant influx of new nurses, a core group provides a continuity of personnel that would otherwise be lacking. Nonetheless, it would be a mistake to overestimate the extent to which any hospital unit, even an intensive care unit, can be a nursing unit.

Nurses, as nearly every observer of the occupation has observed, depend heavily on physicians. Nurses are identified in the organizational charts of most hospitals as part of a distinctive nursing hierarchy, vested with responsibility for the pay, promotions, and work assignments of individual nurses. In this sense, nursing has achieved a measure, albeit limited, of collective self-direction. Yet it is hospital administrators, many of whom are physicians, very few of whom are nurses, who set the broad parameters of nursing, who determine what is nursing's proper place and what is the physician's. Moreover, it is individual physicians—who are officially part of an entirely different hierarchy from nurses—who order the bulk of the therapies and procedures that make up the daily workload of the hospital nurse. In this sense, nursing is, at least organizationally, a subordinate occupation.

The organizational subordination of nurses should not, however, be confused with what might be called the cultural subordination of nursing. Although nurses may be bound organizationally (and to some extent legally) to follow doctors' orders, they are not bound, save for their own inclinations, to agree with those orders or the logic that underlies them. Indeed, it is precisely the possibility that nurses orient themselves to medical care in a manner significantly different from doctors that is the basis for claims that they can be effective advocates for the patients in their care.

The potential for disagreement between nurses and doctors is exacerbated by the differences in the backgrounds of recruits to the two occupations. Not only are nurses almost exclusively women and doctors predominantly men, but also nurses differ from doctors in class origin and religious background. At both Outerboro and Countryside, the doctors are disproportionately Jewish and, even more heavily, upper middle class in origin. In contrast, the nursing staff at both hospitals is disproportionately Catholic and, modally, lower middle class in origin.

The relationship between doctors and nurses is, then, one fraught with the potential for conflict. In some situations, doctors and nurses may avoid conflict simply by avoiding each other. But in intensive care, the critical condition of patients and the constant presence of both doctors and nurses magnify their dependence on each other. Unable to escape each other, neither can they escape conflict.

Many doctors, particularly at Countryside, offer high praise for ICU nurses: "by far the best in the hospital," "fantastic," "a pleasure to work with." But they are also, particularly at Outerboro, acutely aware that their good relations with the nursing staff are fragile. To some, problems with the nurses result from nothing more systematic than clashes of personality. ICU nurses, they claim, are "prima donnas," "callous," or "downright obnoxious." But conflicts between doctors and nurses, as other physicians recognize, run deeper. "It's hard dealing with the ICU nurses," one Outerboro resident told me, "because they have a sort of territorial feeling about [the unit]. They're there all the time, and they have a way of doing things. They can really push you around if you let them." "We were arresting [resuscitating] a patient," another resident told me,

and the nurse was worried that the containers . . . were placed on the bed. She wanted to know who made this mess, not "Why are you pumping on this patient's chest?" It's like, "Who made the mess?" because their task . . . is to keep the bed clean. Ours at that point was to keep this woman alive.

These are conflicts over authority and responsibility, over priorities and the division of labor.

While the ICU physicians balance their criticism of ICU nurses with praise, the ICU nurses—particularly at Outerboro—are often more strident in their criticism of ICU physicians. If physicians think that their own decisions are the critical ones, nurses see themselves as the front line of medical care. Above all, they often feel that their efforts on that front line are not appreciated:

So basically we have the patient's life in our hands. I mean, you can give orders all you want. If somebody doesn't do it, what good is it? I think the nurses have a lot to do with the patients' care and the total outcome. Like we had Mr. Listell and his leg, I don't know if you remember, his leg had no pulse and so [one doctor] was congratulating [another doctor]. "You saved his leg." I started to laugh. I said to myself, "We were the ones that saw that the guy had no pulse." . . . If you tell somebody to do this and they don't do it, you aren't going to get any results. I think the nurses, the final outcome depends upon the care that we give.

Well, they can sit in the back and write orders all day and all night and if those orders aren't picked up, then nothing gets done for the patient. . . . But they sit back there and make decisions, but they don't do squat, basically, about getting things done. That's why it's my antidoctor week again, so this is not good. When they sit around taking credit, a lot of the times, for how well you did and sometimes when you sit there and you try to discuss with them about the patients and they'll say, "We'll do this and we'll do that," but they don't do anything. They basically sit back there and make the decisions. They have basically no contact with the patient as an individual. . . . Early in the morning they draw their bloods, they listen to their lungs, they listen to their bellies, maybe chitchat a bit, and the only other times they're back in there usually is to start an IV or to draw blood.

If the nurses resent physicians in general, they are particularly resentful of the new interns and residents whom, in the character of a teaching hospital, they confront—and often help train—every year. An Outerboro nurse:

Well, sometimes I feel as though they're here two weeks twice a year. I do the same damn thing every single day for years and years and years. You see the same things. Certain things happen. Patient drops his pressure, you jack up the dopamine. You can't just shut the dopamine off; you've got to bring it down slowly, because this is the way it is. You learn after a while. . . . You know how much a patient is going to react. Some doctors come over and they just push the pump down twenty drops and you've got a pressure of fifty again. That sometimes drives me out of my mind because, from experience, all this comes. When you've been here a while, you have that experience which they don't have.

A Countryside nurse put it simply: "I'd like us to get more respect from the doctors. I'd like the doctors to be less arrogant."

At Countryside, a few of the intensive care nurses play what some observers have called "the doctor-nurse game," subtly manipulating physicians while avoiding open conflict and making a show of support.[6] "Your presentation," Marianne told me, "is the key. . . . If you come on like gangbusters with these people, forget it. They aren't going to listen to a word, especially . . . Ken. . . . But if you use some degree of diplomacy . . . I think that they are very open." But the "doctor-nurse game" only masks conflict. It does not eliminate it. "If they start giving me problems," Marianne continued, "then I tend to get my feathers ruffled. I won't make it easy for them." In dealing with "arrogant" housestaff who would not let "the nurse make any decisions about anything," she had a well-developed strategy:

6. Leonard Stein, "The Doctor-Nurse Game," *Archives of General Psychiatry* 16 (1967): 669–702; Leonard Stein, David Watts, and Timothy Howell, "The Doctor-Nurse Game Revisited," *New England Journal of Medicine* 322 (1990): 546–49.

Any labs I get, I will call them. Whereas the others, I will just call them with something significant. But I will stay on a case and say, "You want to do this this way, we'll do it this way." And I go right down the line. I'm strict according to all the rules. Makes them crazy after a while. But they learn. They end up, I get the message. Then you do back off.

At Outerboro, conflict is more explicit. There, the nurses do not bear their resentments silently. Doctors and nurses trade barbs nearly every day, blunting them only slightly with a frequently bantering tone. (For example, as a nurse, conducting an orientation for a group of new nurses, prepared to battle a group of rounding doctors over a bedside chart, one doctor joked to another, "She's teaching them how to be uncooperative.") At least twice I saw the conflicts between nurses and doctors erupt into open shouting matches: once when a nurse interrupted rounds to complain that a patient had thrown a clipboard at her, once over whether a nurse would accompany a patient outside the unit for a procedure on a day when the nurses were short staffed. Whatever the situation elsewhere, the nurses in the Outerboro ICU do not shirk from open disagreement with physicians.

What, though, are we to make of these disagreements? It is one thing to say that nurses criticize doctors. This will come as no surprise to anyone who has taken the time to speak to even a few nurses. It is, however, quite a different thing to say that these criticisms are based on high principle or that they represent different orientations to patient care. At Outerboro and Countryside, they do not. Noisily at Outerboro, in somewhat more muted tones at Countryside, the nurses are critical of physicians, but for their treatment of nurses, not for their treatment of patients. On matters of patient care, they are remarkably quiet.

Consider Claire and Angela.

Claire is virtually unique among the Outerboro ICU nurses. Just having finished a master's degree, she readily invoked nursing theory, nursing professionalism, and patient advocacy. Claire suggested a broad role for nursing:

I think there should be involvement of nursing in every step of the process. . . . I think they're good about handing tasks out here because they don't like to do them. But they're not really good about taking what nursing has to tell them and involve them later in the plan. . . . Nursing as a patient advocate has to air the patient's views. I think that's very disconcerting to physicians, who think that nurses are then being belligerent when they are supporting the patient's views.

At the core of the notion of the nurse as advocate is an expectation that nurses, because they provide hands-on care, know patients and their families

better than do doctors. Like other ICU nurses, Claire stressed that nurses
know patients in ways the physicians do not. The physician, she told me,

doesn't have to be in there turning him every two hours. He doesn't have to be in there
cleaning up his diarrhea. I think that's really hard. So not only is their stint short;
during the day they're able to get back from it more. They work really, really hard, but
I think it's easier to get less involved, not even attached to the patient.

Claire was particularly critical of the physicians' failure to involve nurses
in decisions to limit treatment, to issue what are known as "Do Not Resuscitate" orders. Moreover, she articulates a distinctive nursing point of view
on that decision. The doctors, she complained, "never really have to deal
with the fact that the patient is dying and they can just write the orders."
Concerned with the patient's comfort, with care rather than cure, she sees
herself (and other nurses as well) as less willing than the physicians to subject
patients to extended and often painful treatments.[7]

A nurse may have had discussions with the family. A nurse may have had discussions
with the patient. A nurse knows the torture the patient is going through and can give
at least the patient's reaction to it in terms of resistance, in terms of depression, in
terms of all these things which I think are overlooked. I think a nurse has to be
brought in on it—how the nurse feels about it, but more so from the patient's point of
view.

Claire, then, sees the nurse as something more than a technician. She
complained that the doctors often see nurses as "mini-interns," failing to
recognize that nursing knowledge is not simply a pale imitation of doctors'
knowledge but something altogether distinctive.

I don't think they really understand what nurses do even in ICU. I don't think they
understand that it does matter to me that the pillow is pulled out from underneath my
patient, that how I organize my care makes a difference in how this patient does
during the day, [that] whether he's interrupted every thirty minutes or every two hours
makes a difference. I don't think that any at all understand that.

Even more, Claire stressed, the nurse's organizational role provides her with
privileged access to matters that physicians can only guess at. "How the pa-

7. There is a conventional wisdom that nurses are likelier than physicians to object to limiting the treatment of terminally ill patients. In fact, they are less likely to object. The mispercep-
tion results from the consequences of cases in which nurses do object. Such cases have become
the basis for occasional legal actions and scandals while objections on the other side (to continued treatment) go unnoticed. Similar findings appear in Anspach, "Prognostic Conflict," in
Jeanne Harley Guillemin and Linda Lytle Holmstrom, *Mixed Blessings: Intensive Care for Newborns* (New York: Oxford University Press, 1986), both studies of neonatal intensive care units,
and in Wolf's study of a general nursing ward in an acute care hospital reported in *Nurses' Work*.

tient is doing, not only in a physical realm in terms of their bodily secretions and everything, but maybe in how they and their family are coping, how the patient is coping, what the patient desires." According to Claire, then, the nurse is a patient advocate, with her advocacy rooted in both a distinctive body of technical knowledge and a distinctive role in the hospital division of labor. At the same time, the nurse is an advocate for a distinctive set of values, more concerned with the patient as a person, less narrowly focused on laboratory findings and physiology than is the physician.

Claire is not alone. A few nurses—more at Countryside than at Outerboro—voice all or part of the same concerns. But these nurses are a minority. They are of interest not so much as examples of what nursing is but as examples of what nursing might aspire to.

Angela is far more typical. She had been working in the Outerboro ICU for four years when I interviewed her. She had transferred to the ICU, after eight years on a medical ward, because "I just felt I was getting too involved and I wanted to change, not that you don't get involved with some of the patients in the ICU. It's just a little more difficult. I think you can put more of a barrier up." Angela is milder and more qualified in her criticism of physicians than are most of the other unit nurses: "I respect them a lot. I think they know a lot. . . . For the most part I think a lot will listen to you. Some won't, just absolutely won't." "You need," she suggested, "give and take of both parts." But it is not at all clear what Angela means to give.

Like Claire, Angela could imagine a distinctive voice for nurses as advocates for comfort and care rather than for aggressive treatment and cure. But she has not, as she suggested in discussing one case—a woman who had lingered in the ICU for many months while dying of esophageal cancer—pushed hard for those views in practice: "Maybe more input should have been done into even making her comfortable or putting her on methadone or doing something. Maybe we're guilty of this, too. Maybe we the nurses should have done something more to push, some more comfort measures." Unlike Claire, but like most of the other ICU nurses, Angela does not see it as her place to take part in discussions of whether to make a patient DNR ("Do Not Resuscitate"): "We can give our input, and they'll have to listen to us or just hear what we have to say. But I think it's more the decision of the doctors and the families, more so than what we have to say."

The differences between Claire and Angela extend also to questions of what and how much to tell patients and their families. According to Claire, nurses have a special role in talking to patients. "I think a lot of families are very calmed down by telling them the overall, how the patient is doing.

That's all they need. They need to know how they slept, what their fever is like, those kinds of things. . . . I think that a nurse can do a lot."

In contrast, Angela, again speaking for a majority of the ICU nurses, recognizes that she probably should spend more time talking to patients and their families, but acknowledges that she in fact does not: "You feel that you're working a lot, you're doing all of these technical things, the machines, the respirators, and the family is sort of by the wayside." Because she claims no special knowledge of the patient, neither does Angela see any issues of principled difference from physicians in what to tell patients.

Usually I would like to know what the doctors are telling the families first and then hopefully they're telling them truthful situations, what's going on, the prognosis, and just trying to, I'll try to, if they don't understand, just support what the doctor has said and try to explain it in easier terms.

I pressed her: "Would you *ever* tell a patient a prognosis or a diagnosis if the doctor hadn't?" "I don't know," she answered. "That's touchy. I don't know what to say about that." I pressed on: "Can you think of a time when you have?"

Angela: I can think of a time in the past when I was on [the ward], out of the unit, when a young woman was dying of cancer and the attending refused to tell and the husband didn't want her to know and they were all playing this charade. I remember it was horrible. I'm giving her morphine injections and telling her it was bronchial dilate and this sort of thing. I don't think the woman was really fooled. I don't like that.
RZ: So you went ahead and told her?
Angela: No. We never, we didn't, but we all felt really bad about it.

What, then, does Angela think should be up to nurses? Her first answer was vague. "Maybe just input into the type of care, the quality of care the patients get." But even when asked to be more specific, all Angela could think of was "maybe weaning a patient from a respirator, that sort of thing." This is not the counsel of an angel of mercy, or of a patient advocate. It is the counsel of a technician.

The Limits of Nursing

Let me be more systematic. Nurses, as both Claire and Angela suggest, do have a distinctive perspective on patient care. They are more concerned than physicians with comfort and emotional adjustments to illness, less concerned with cure. But this perspective does not make nurses angels of mercy. Neither does it provide nurses with an effective basis for patient advocacy. Rather, it becomes little more than the grounds on which nurses attempt, with only limited success, to differentiate their technical skills from those of physicians.

First, although ICU nurses are more concerned than ICU physicians with the emotional life of their patients (and their patients' families), this concern is distinctly bounded. "They need the emotional support of their family," one Countryside nurse acknowledged of her patients. But, she continued, "I am their nurse. . . . I can't be their family too."

I get the family involved as much as I can. Maybe not in the hands-on kind of care. But I let them know that I am doing this part, the technical part, and I am also supportive to this patient. But I am not the husband, sister, wife, whatever.

Nurses do, in the hospital division of labor, have more hands-on involvement with patients than do physicians. And it is nurses, rather than physicians, who are usually the first to answer calls for help and the only ones to arrange pillows. Yet even these differences should not be exaggerated. Hands-on involvement is not necessarily converted to emotional involvement or a personal relationship. One Countryside nurse, for example, claimed "I know my patients better" than do nurses on general floors. "We do things differently here." She continued:

We get to look at patients in more invasive ways and more intimate ways than anybody else. All the anatomy and physiology and everything else that you learn becomes more real. It's not abstract. You get to actually see the science at work and how it works.

What it means to "know [her] patients better" or to know them in "more intimate ways," then, is not to know their hopes and fears, to feel for them in special ways. It is to know their "anatomy and physiology."

The absence of a strong orientation to the emotional life of patients is, in part, a matter of choice among ICU nurses. Like Angela, many nurses prefer the ICU precisely because it allows them to avoid personal relationships with their patients. It would be a mistake, however, to attribute the lack of emotional involvement simply to choice. Some nurses do seek more personal relationships with patients and families. "The technical things," one Countryside nurse told me, "are too routine."

I like to spend time with family in the room, with the patient, too. Have that total interaction thing. That's the part that makes you feel good, seeing that you've done something for the family, seeing that you've done something for the patient. That's what makes you feel good at the end of the day. . . . It's not getting a Swan in.

But even for those nurses who are inclined to get more involved with their patients, the structure of the unit and the character of its patients do not permit it. In part, this is a matter of priorities. "Sometimes you can get wrapped up in the technical aspect of doing labs or getting a bunch of numbers," a Countryside nurse observed. "A lot of times its hard to see the patient through all the tubes and meds." "Unfortunately," another lamented,

when you are prioritizing, your patient's needs come first. And around here patient needs means technical first. Then you are allowed to go into more social psychological. Your priorities always have to be square in your mind. There are times I've had families falling apart, and its been so busy with my patient trying to keep them alive that unfortunately that family gets lost in the wind.[8]

In part, it is a matter of scheduling. Not only are the nurses "on" less than every other day; there is no systematic attempt to see that they cover the same patients when they are on for consecutive days.[9] Consider, for example, the pattern of nursing coverage for Lewis Hammer, a more or less typical Countryside patient, as shown in figure 5.1. In eight days, over fifteen shifts, ten different nurses provided coverage. Even when the unit makes a special effort, as they did for Kelly Connors, whom I introduced briefly in chapter 2, there are significant discontinuities in nursing care, as shown in figure 5.2. Over twenty-five days, covering forty-nine shifts, no fewer than twenty-one different nurses covered Kelly, none for more than eight shifts, ten for only one. With this pattern of nursing coverage added to the rapid turnover of patients in the ICU, nurses (like physicians) are often caring for patients they have never seen before. I asked one nurse how much she knew about a patient she was caring for on the day I interviewed her. "Little to nothing. Basically the report I got was very sketchy, and I just kind of glanced at . . . the intern's admission notes just to see the past history on him, but that's really all I know." Even when patients have been in the unit for an extended stay, the nurses may not get to know them well: "Like Mr. Finn who has been

8. Wolf observes that the nurses she studied in an acute care hospital had a narrow view even of what was technically efficacious: "They viewed the efficacy of medications in a magical or unexplainable way and often did not consider the possibility that other care-giving actions . . . could have been responsible for improvement in a patient's condition." *Nurses' Work*, p. 180.

9. For an analysis of the difference between nursing schedules and doctors' schedules, see Eviatar Zerubavel, *Patterns of Time in Hospital Life* (Chicago: University of Chicago Press, 1979), especially pp. 54–59.

here for God knows how long, even though this is the first day I've taken care of him. I have never caught rounds on him at all, so his whole story I have no idea about."

Although the nurses themselves may be more concerned with care than are the physicians, they nonetheless accept the physicians' conception that

	Day Shift	Night Shift
Day 1	Nurse A	Nurse B
Day 2	Nurse C	Nurse D
Day 3	Nurse E	Nurse D
Day 4	Nurse E	Nurse F
Day 5	Nurse G	Nurse F
Day 6	Nurse H	Nurse F
Day 7	Nurse I	Nurse J
Day 8	Nurse I	

Figure 5.1. Pattern of nursing shifts, Lewis Hammer.

	Day Shift	Night Shift
Day 1		Nurse A
Day 2	Nurse B	Nurse C
Day 3	Nurse B	Nurse D
Day 4	Nurse E	Nurse D
Day 5	Nurse E	Nurse F
Day 6	Nurse G	Nurse D
Day 7	Nurse H	Nurse I
Day 8	Nurse E	Nurse J
Day 9	Nurse J	Nurse K
Day 10	Nurse L	Nurse K
Day 11	Nurse M	Nurse D
Day 12	Nurse I	Nurse M
Day 13	Nurse I	Nurse N
Day 14	Nurse N	Nurse O
Day 15	Nurse P	Nurse Q
Day 16	Nurse P	Nurse D
Day 17	Nurse N	Nurse D
Day 18	Nurse N	Nurse I
Day 19	Nurse R	Nurse I
Day 20	Nurse R	Nurse I
Day 21	Nurse S	Nurse T
Day 22	Nurse N	Nurse T
Day 23	Nurse U	Nurse T
Day 24	Nurse R	Nurse I
Day 25	Nurse N	Nurse I

Figure 5.2. Pattern of nursing shifts, Kelly Connors.

the unit as a whole is more concerned with cure. Nowhere is this more evident than in the nurses' orientation to long-term unit patients. If the nurses were, in fact, "angels of mercy," they would be as interested in these patients as in any others. Yet no more than physicians do the nurses welcome patients who linger. At Countryside, where the ICU includes both surgical and medical patients, virtually all of the nurses prefer the former, precisely because they are in and out of the unit quickly, because results are visible.

We prefer surgical patients . . . because their problems are more easily identifiable and more easily correctable. . . . And you can see the results. It's a measurable, tangible thing. The patient comes in Tuesday, you treat a, b, and c. On Friday they are starting to get better . . . and you get them transferred. Medical patients, they get better, they get worse, they get better.

Rather than treating dying patients—patients beyond cure but no less in need of care—as part of their special calling, nurses join physicians in a view of such patients as inappropriate to the ICU. As the head nurse at Outerboro told me while discussing two patients whose deaths were preceded by long unit stays, "They just need an alternate level of care. They just need to be someplace where they can be maintained on the ventilator."

Second, the ICU nurses at Outerboro and Countryside are not patient advocates. Nurses may explain procedures to patients in more detail than do physicians. But they do not break the silence of physicians to inform patients of diagnoses or prognoses. This is more or less official policy. According to Outerboro's head nurse, "Having been in situations where a lot of what you say is misinterpreted by the family, I'd rather not have the nurses get involved." Linda Goodwin, the head nurse at Countryside, expressed similar sentiments. Nurses, she suggested, are "obligated to be as frank and as open as possible" with patients and their families. Moreover, she claimed, "nurses can sometimes take what the doctor says and bring it down to a layman-type level and sometimes the doctor can't do that." But, she acknowledged, there are, from time to time, physicians "who will be very specific that [they] don't want the family to know" about a grim prognosis. And in these instances she hoped that "the nurse would abide by [the physician's] wishes. . . . It should come from the physician if it's prognosis. . . . I would like to see the physician be the first one to talk to the family." And even Claire conceded that "telling a client a diagnosis is the physician's responsibility."

Because nurses are unwilling—or unable—to discuss diagnosis and prognosis, it is also difficult for them to raise critical issues with patients or their families except in very general terms. Josie, for example, one of the more aggressive Countryside nurses, explained that she would sometimes raise issues that doctors had not. "I will prepare the family, when a patient comes in and if it doesn't look good. I will say to them, in my patient teaching, I will talk to them about a trach [a tracheostomy], a future trach down the line, because a patient can only be on a ventilator for a certain period of time." But even Josie's efforts are tentative and cautious. "I try to teach them," she quickly conceded, "in a general way that this is what happens and this might be. And I always ask what has the doctor told them first. And I always try to reiterate that."

Asking a dying patient's family to consider a Do Not Resuscitate order or attempting to obtain a reluctant patient's consent for a procedure requires a discussion of possible outcomes, outcomes that nurses are not equipped to specify. As a result, most nurses do even less than Josie. As one put it, echoing Angela's views, "I've never discussed with anyone what they would want their arrest status to be. . . . I don't think it's my position." "That's too much responsibility," another suggested. "I can't make decisions for myself, never mind for somebody else."

Neither is this a matter of nurses maintaining a united front to patients while lobbying behind the scenes. To be sure, a few nurses (especially at Countryside) will make suggestions to physicians. But they rarely assert their views with any great insistence.[10] Although nurses at both Outerboro and Countryside attend rounds regularly, they typically do not speak up unless invited to by a physician. And when nurses do speak up, it is most often to offer information about such matters as secretions, medications, respiration, or the patient's wakefulness. Not once during rounds at either hospital did I hear a nurse suggest that a patient should be told more than he or she had already been told by physicians. Only twice at Outerboro and less than a half dozen times at Countryside did I hear nurses question a patient's resuscitation status, and then (with one exception) only to *ask* for clarifications of what that status was.

Third, whatever anyone else might hope for, more than anything else nurses themselves value—and are valued for—their technical skills. A Countryside nurse reflected on her own priorities in training new recruits to the unit:

10. Wolf makes a similar observation: "The nurses thought they knew certain areas of health care better than doctors, other hospital personnel, family members, and patients. However, nurses' defensive response to the behaviors of those who invaded their turf remained largely rhetorical. Although they dealt daily with those 'invaders,' they seldom confronted them face-to-face." *Nurses' Work*, p. 254.

You're definitely trained with the technical skills, and that is the heart of orientation. That is orientation. When I orient somebody, I teach them how to put a Swan in, how to put an A line in, how to do this, this drug does that—that kind of stuff. I hope during orientation that, as a role model, . . . they can stand back and see my interactions and use me as a teaching tool. . . . But there's nothing as set, pat, . . . to the interpersonal relationships.

"I think they tend to be real technically oriented here," an Outerboro nurse told me.

Like, the nurse who you're giving this patient to is going to be more concerned about whether you change dressings, not whether you let the patient sleep, for example, which they get none of. Or you had a big conversation with a patient and the patient really needed to vent something. They're not going to really worry about that. They're going to worry about whether everything's dated properly, was this changed because it's twenty-four hours now, it has to be changed. Those kinds of things.

It is by virtue of their technical skills that nurses win the respect of physicians. While the Outerboro and Countryside doctors are more or less indifferent to the nurses' emotional skills and often surprised at the suggestion that they might participate in critical decisions—"What role would they play?" one resident asked—they very much appreciate nurses' knowledge of procedures. "They know where all the tubes go," one Outerboro resident told me. "That's important. . . . They sense when something's wrong, or they'll notice a new sign, and most often it comes from the nurses. That's where we get our physical exam data." "They know how to use and give more medications than any other nurses I ever heard of," a Countryside intern added.

They know how to use Swans. They know how to hook up a monitor. They know whole different spectrums of medical problems. They know about people in DKA [diabetic ketoacidosis]. They know about people in DIC [disseminated intravascular coagulation]. . . . They know all that stuff. They are much more sophisticated.

Nurses earn respect from physicians insofar as they are able to help complete the technical tasks that are the stock in trade of the physicians themselves.

At the same time, it is in terms of technical skills—not patient advocacy or a distinctive commitment to care rather than cure—that nurses make their strongest claims against physicians and express, however faintly, their most principled criticisms of patient care. Elements of these criticisms are found in Claire's insistence that doctors don't really understand what nurses do. They are also apparent in Angela's wish that physicians would consult with her before weaning a patient from a respirator. But they are perhaps most apparent in the constantly reiterated claim that nurses train physicians:

Even the resident, she had only put in a couple of Swans in her internship year, so she said, "Now what do I do?" When you've seen it time after time after time, again, it's a technical thing. "Yes, this gets plugged into here and you do this." . . . It has to be handled kind of gently. You don't want to step on anybody's ego but, and that's a big reason too why there's a lot of breakdown.

Technical skill, unlike patient advocacy or a commitment to care, earns the nurses a measure of respect. Doctors, one Outerboro nurse complained, "don't give us the respect that we deserve." But she had also seen a change in the unit over the previous year and a half:

Before I felt we had no decision-making powers. Now I feel like we have a lot more because we're doing all the hemodynamics and drawing bloods and total evaluation of the patient, which makes you more reliable than when you walk up to a doctor and say, "Well, the patient's short of breath but I don't know what the ABG [arterial blood gas] is because I can't draw it." You're able to say what things are and show them that you are confident. Then they take you more seriously.

The unit's head nurse struck a similar theme. "I'm somebody," she told me, "who feels that nursing as a practice in general should be allowed almost total autonomy." To earn this autonomy, she proposed turning over to her staff more and more of what are currently the technical responsibilities of physicians:

I'm going to tell you quite honestly, the thing that I'm currently having typed up is a procedure and protocol for nurses here to start cardioverting and defibrillating patients. They don't currently do that here for many reasons. . . . I don't want them to necessarily get into arrhythmia diagnosing and determine that this person is in V-tach when in fact it may not be. . . . I think the fact that somebody can put two paddles on a patient and hit the buttons, I think that's a different task. I think the nurses can do that. The reason I want the nurses to do that is because I have many different pieces of equipment here. The housestaff who rotate through two weeks at a time are less familiar with the equipment than the nurses. So just for efficacy's sake to have the nurses do it is better. But after that I would seriously consider looking at the nurses putting in arterial lines, systemic arterial lines.

Not patient advocacy, not a special relationship to patients, but the right to "put two paddles" on a patient in cardiac arrest or to place a line monitoring blood flow leads the way to autonomy. This is a strategy with deep roots in nursing history and nursing practice but also one with severe limitations.

Ever since Florence Nightingale helped establish modern nursing through her heroic efforts in the Crimean War, nursing leadership has emphasized technical skill as a means of differentiating nurses from their potential competitors. For Nightingale, an emphasis on technical skill was a means of differentiating the "professional nurse" from the women of often questionable character and from the well-intentioned but untrained nuns who provided much of the care for the hospitalized sick through the middle of the nineteenth century. For succeeding generations of nursing leaders in the United States, an emphasis on technical skills acquired through formal education seemed to join nurses to the "professional project" that has provided one important route to collective mobility in this country.[11]

To be sure, some observers have suggested that rank and file nurses have never endorsed their leadership's emphasis on technical skill as the distinctive virtue of their occupation. But in the ICU, there are some special incentives for doing so. Above all, by emphasizing technical skills, the ICU nurses not only distinguish themselves from the large number of technicians and therapists of lesser skill who populate the contemporary hospital, but also from other nurses. Because the intensive care nurses are selected from already experienced nurses, must complete a special course, and are permitted to perform a broader range of procedures than "floor" nurses, they think of themselves, one nurse told me, as "an elite." Another added:

I enjoy the independence that we have here with the work that we do, the fact that we're able to do so much more than the regular nurses on the floor. The status that goes behind being an ICU nurse, the doctors respect you a lot more. You find that on the floor they really don't respect you as much. Here they require more knowledge and we are able to use that knowledge.

For the ICU nurses an emphasis on technical skills ensures a more successful claim to high status than would an emphasis on patient advocacy or a special devotion to care.

But once having entered a logic of hierarchy the nurses find it hard to escape. This is the fundamental dilemma of nursing ideology. If nurses emphasize their technical skills in order to establish their priority over therapists and technicians or, in the ICU, their priority over other nurses, the very same claim ensures that they will defer to physicians.

Nurses do have technical skills that doctors do not. They know how to formulate nursing plans, to "deliver" medications, to sit a patient up, to clean a wound. Moreover, they do, as they claim, "train" new interns. But neither of these sets of skills involves nurses in the core tasks of diagnosis and prognosis that are the basis for long-term planning. That, they freely acknowl-

11. Melosh, *Physician's Hand;* Reverby, *Ordered.*

edge, is the proper domain of the physician. Having made claims of technical expertise for themselves, they are ill equipped to challenge the technical expertise of physicians on the central issues of what to tell a patient or how aggressively to treat.

The emphasis on technical skills rather than the emotional side of nursing is, in large part, a matter of choice—both collectively as a strategy of professional mobility and individually as an expression of personal preferences. But it is not simply a matter of choice. It is technical skill—not empathy or a special faculty for kindness—that is recognized and rewarded by physicians and by a hospital hierarchy. Nurses may concern themselves with care rather than cure, with the social and emotional aspects of illness rather than physiology, but in the ICU they are rarely able to express that concern

Nurses, Claire's disclaimer notwithstanding, have become "mini-interns." They are not patient advocates. They are not "angels of mercy." Like physicians, they have become technicians.

6

Patienthood and the Culture of Rights

As if in a magic trick, the patient vanishes, hidden behind machines and tubes, there unseen by doctors and nurses. But as in any good magic trick, the patient also reappears. Only, in intensive care the patient reappears not simply in another place—on the wings of the stage or at the back of an auditorium—but in an altogether different form. In particular, the patient reappears not as a distinctive personality so much as the more or less abstract embodiment of rights. This, too, has an element of illusion.

The notion of rights in medical care (as distinct from rights to medical care) emerges out of the predominantly technical orientation of contemporary medicine. It is made possible and sustained by the very impersonality of the doctor-patient relationship. Yet most discussions of the notion of rights have focused on it as a narrowly legal, not as a more generally social, concept. As a result, most discussions of rights in medicine have focused on legal doctrine, particularly the doctrine of informed consent. But as I will argue, the direct effects of informed consent as a legal doctrine are limited in intensive care. In contrast, a notion of rights as a broad cultural concept (the acceptance of which is among the indirect effects of the legal doctrine) has had far-reaching consequences, including, most important, an empowerment of the patient and, in some circumstances, the patient's family.

Informed Consent as Legal Doctrine

The legal doctrine of informed consent was first formulated by a California court in 1957 and has since been elaborated through both a long series of malpractice cases and legislative actions in all but three states.[1] Put simply,

1. President's Commission for the Study of Ethical Problems in Medicine and Biomedical and Behavioral Research, *Making Health Care Decisions*, vol. 3: *Studies on the Foundations of Informed Consent* (Washington, DC: Government Printing Office, 1982), pp. 193–251. See also Jay Katz, *The Silent World of Doctor and Patient* (New York: Free Press, 1984); Ruth R. Faden and

informed consent is intended to enable patients to make decisions about their own medical care by requiring physicians to provide them with sufficient information about the risks and benefits of treatments and procedures as well as about alternatives to any proposed treatment or procedure. In New York, for example, a provision of the general Public Health Law now requires that physicians inform patients of "any reasonably foreseeable risks" before obtaining consent. Moreover, even in many states without legislation containing specific provisions about informed consent, the doctrine is now well established. Thus, in Massachusetts, one of the states without such legislation, courts have required that physicians provide patients with "all significant medical information . . . material to an intelligent decision by the patient." [2] Informed consent does not—and is not intended to—allow patients to demand particular treatments. However, it is intended, at least in principle, to assure patients the right to refuse treatment. It is the primary expression of the emphasis on autonomy and self-determination that permeates much of contemporary medical ethics.

In practice, the situation is significantly different. As a specifically legal doctrine, informed consent presupposes a model of decision making that has little to do with the realities of medical care. As Lidz, Meisel, and their colleagues have observed, in their important empirical study of informed consent, "Law's vision of medical decisionmaking involves an implicit assumption . . . that medical practice is discrete—that is, broken into distinct parts, or decision units—and that there can be consent by the patient to each of these individual parts." [3] In fact, medical practice, especially in intensive care, is far more of a continuous process. Each treatment or procedure typically depends on a prior treatment or procedure and implies a subsequent treatment or procedure. Informed consent, then, requires of physicians a style of thought (and explanation) radically different from that to which they are accustomed.

Tom L. Beauchamp, *A History and Theory of Informed Consent* (New York: Oxford University Press, 1986).

2. President's Commission, *Making Health Care Decisions*, vol. 3, pp. 230, 222.

3. Charles W. Lidz and Alan Meisel with Janice L. Holden, John H. Marx, and Mark Munetz, "Informed Consent and the Structure of Medical Care," in President's Commission for the Study of Ethical Problems in Medicine and Biomedical and Behavioral Research, *Making Health Care Decisions*, vol. 2: *Appendices, Empirical Studies of Informed Consent* (Washington, DC: Government Printing Office, 1982), p. 401. See also Charles Lidz, Alan Meisel, Eviatar Zerubavel, Mary Carter, Regina Sestak, and Loren Roth, *Informed Consent* (New York: Guilford Press, 1984); Charles Lidz, Alan Meisel, Marian Osterweis, Janice L. Holden, John H. Marx, and Mark Munetz, "Barriers to Informed Consent," *Annals of Internal Medicine* 1983 (99): 539–43.

Moreover, as Lidz and Meisel concluded after extensive fieldwork and interviews, most patients simply "are not interested in, nor do they believe themselves capable of, playing the role assigned by law."[4] In intensive care, the very disability of patients diminishes yet further the number of patients who invoke their right to refuse treatment.

Even when a patient does, at first, refuse a treatment, physicians and nurses may persist until that patient finally consents. And in most states (including New York and Massachusetts), even when the patient is adamant in refusing treatments, the law recognizes a number of exceptions to the general requirement of informed consent: most importantly, instances of emergency or incompetence. In intensive care, however, in the face of acute illness, neither emergency nor incompetence is so much an exception as the general rule.

The result of all this is that informed consent plays only a small role in the units at Countryside and Outerboro. Over the course of my research, only six patients at Countryside explicitly refused treatments or procedures recommended by their doctors. But even this total is an overstatement. Two of the cases are ambiguous. One involved a woman who refused an endoscopy, a procedure the ICU staff favored but that her private physician may have recommended against. The other involved a ninety-two-year-old woman who refused intubation because, in her words, she had already "had a full life," a decision and rationale the ICU staff greeted with admiration despite their having suggested the procedure. In two more cases relatively healthy patients signed themselves out of the hospital against medical advice. Short of forcibly restraining them, the unit physicians would have been hard put to prevent them from leaving. It is unlikely that these cases would have been handled differently in the absence of the doctrine of informed consent. In a fifth case, that of a man who refused placement of a Swan-Ganz catheter, the ICU staff inserted the catheter anyway, justifying their action by invoking the patient's "varying mental status" and the agreement of the patient's family with their course of action. In the sixth case, that of a woman who refused reintubation, the ICU staff did respect the patient's wishes. But even in this case, they did so reluctantly and only after having agreed among themselves to reintubate if the patient's respiratory condition worsened (which it did not).

At Outerboro, the situation was little different. Over the course of my research, eight patients refused treatments or procedures recommended by

4. Lidz et al., "Informed Consent," p. 404.

physicians. But in four of these cases, the patients later changed their minds
under pressure from the ICU physicians as well as, in some cases, their own
families. In only one of the remaining four cases—that of a woman who
refused intubation—did the ICU staff honor the request. In the other three,
the ICU staff went ahead with treatment, each time justifying their action by
invoking both the altered mental status of the patient and a notion of responsibility quite different from that implicit in the doctrine of informed consent.
Mr. Andrews, for example, a man in his thirties with a presumptive (but un-
confirmed) diagnosis of AIDS, had refused intubation. The night that Andrews was admitted to the unit, his intern documented his refusal thoroughly
in the chart, providing an almost textbook application of the principles of
informed consent:

> I have discussed intubation [with] Pt. He is oriented $\times 3$, and appropriate. He states
> that he has been intubated in the past and that he refuses intubation for any reason
> now. He understands that he has life-threatening illness and may die without intuba-
> tion. He does not want to be intubated for resuscitation if he has [a] pulmonary arrest.
> He feels that he has little to look forward to given his current state of health and does
> not want "to die on a machine." . . . We all feel it is appropriate to respect the pt's
> wishes given his mental state, experience [with] intubation, serious illness, rational
> decision, and full realization of the consequences.

But the following morning, on rounds, the unit attendings overruled the intern's decisions, invoking both the possibility of an AIDS-related mental impairment and a higher responsibility. "The capacity to make a rational decision is restricted," one attending argued, "and we have to step in to act as the
patient's advocate." The other attending was even blunter: "In effect, lie to
him. . . . We have to save his life." Mr. Andrews was intubated immediately
after rounds.

In none of these cases did the physicians see themselves as acting in anything other than the patients' best interests. The physicians were, in the language of medical ethics, more concerned with benevolence than autonomy.
But neither did they see themselves as altogether ignoring autonomy or the
rights of patients. Rather, they ignored a specific refusal in the name of what
they believed to be the larger intention of the patient. Their objection was
not to consent but to the formulation of informed consent as legal doctrine
around the right to refuse a specific treatment.

In practice, then, the relevance of informed consent as a legal doctrine is
distinctly limited in intensive care medicine. It is hardly surprising that, faced
with a legal obligation to describe options in a manner that does little justice
to their complexities and with ample opportunity to ignore patients' treat-

ment refusals, intensive care physicians treat informed consent as little more than a formality. While the ICU physicians at both Outerboro and Countryside do ask their patients to sign official consent forms, they are probably less conscientious in acquiring such signatures than physicians are in other parts of the hospital. And even when they do acquire such signatures, they do so more to meet the letter of the law—to protect themselves and the hospital against the threat of a malpractice suit—than as an occasion to invite the patient to make decisions about his or her own medical care. "Formal informed consent is a legal thing," one resident told me. "I don't see it as an ethical thing. . . . I don't think informed consent exists in an intensive care unit."

The Culture of Rights and the Empowerment of Families

If the notion of rights were limited to informed consent or to legal doctrine, it would merit passing mention as a minor attempt at reform, nothing more. But the notion of rights in medicine is not limited to informed consent or to legal doctrine. It has, rather, since about 1970, become part of the culture of medicine itself. In this sense, the notion of rights does not depend on a specific right of refusal or even on specific decisions. Instead, it involves a very general orientation, of the sort advocated by many medical ethicists, to provide patients direction over the broad purposes of their own medical care. The most important expression of this orientation is a new willingness on the part of physicians to share information with patients.

The evidence for these claims can be found in a wide range of research. Perhaps the single most striking piece of evidence, however, is a 1979 replication of a 1961 study of what physicians tell cancer patients. While, in 1961, 88 percent of physicians reported that they generally did not tell a patient of a cancer diagnosis (and over half that they never or rarely made exceptions to this rule), by 1979 fully 98 percent reported that their general policy was to tell the patient (and two-thirds that they never or rarely made exceptions to *this* rule).[5]

Although little remarked on by most social scientists, there is also considerable evidence that physicians may actually be more inclined to inform pa-

5. Donald Oken, "What to Tell Cancer Patients," *Journal of the American Medical Association* 175 (1961): 1120–28; Dennis H. Novack, Robin Plumer, Raymond L. Smith, Herbert Ochitill, Gary D. Morrow, and John M. Bennett, "Changes in Physicians' Attitudes toward Telling the Cancer Patient," *Journal of the American Medical Association* 241 (1979): 897–900.

tients than patients are to ask for information. For example, a Harris survey, commissioned for the President's Commission for the Study of Ethical Problems in Medicine and Biomedical and Behavioral Research, found that 22 percent of a sample of the general public agreed strongly with the statement that "time spent discussing diagnosis, prognosis, and treatment with patients could be better spent in taking care of patients." In contrast, only 7 percent of a sample of physicians agreed strongly. And, compared to 28 percent of the public sample, over half of the physicians disagreed strongly.[6] Similarly, in a matched sample of patients and physicians drawn from three midwestern states, Haug found that "81% [of physicians] claim views that question physician authority, a higher percentage than the public evidences on the same index."[7] None of this is to say that physicians actually do an effective job of explaining medical conditions to patients. Nor is it to say that physicians always act on their professed beliefs. What is clear, however, is that physicians—as they have not in the past—now recognize at least a basic right of patients to information bearing on their own medical care.

Some of the credit (or blame) for this transformation must surely be assigned to the medical ethics movement—to the cumulative effects of innumerable courses and classes, seminars, conferences, articles, and reports addressing these issues. Some of the credit, too, must surely be assigned to physicians' genuine concern for their patients. But so, too, can at least some of the new recognition of patients' rights be attributed not to a concern for patients but to a distance from them. Consider the remarks of one Outerboro resident:

The easiest thing for a doctor is to present the data to the patient and say "Look, this is what happens. Your life-style might be better with surgery. I can't guarantee it will prolong your life. It might. On the other hand, there is a certain risk." Let him make the decision. The hardest thing you do in medicine is making the decision for a patient and accepting the responsibility of the outcome. That really is a pretty big burden. That is the hardest thing to do, when you talk someone into doing something and it goes wrong. I would love a patient who, I know it is hard, is as informed as I am. . . . People who you have to push a little bit, they are the ones who say, "Doctor, make the decision." I find it to be the hardest. It's hard enough dealing with all the responsibility that you have without having to take on added ones. It really is a heavy

6. Louis Harris and Associates, "Views of Informed Consent and Decisionmaking: Parallel Surveys of Physicians and the Public," in President's Commission for the Study of Ethical Problems in Medicine and Biomedical and Behavioral Research, *Making Health Care Decisions*, vol. 2: *Appendices, Empirical Studies of Informed Consent* (Washington, DC: Government Printing Office, 1982), pp. 17–314.

7. Marie R. Haug and Bebe Lavin, "Practitioner or Patient—Who's in Charge?" *Journal of Health and Social Behavior* 22 (1981): 212–29.

burden. I'm not too crazy about the patient who comes in and says, "I don't want to know anything. I don't want to find out. Doctor, you just take care of me." He puts the whole burden on your shoulders.

In this sense, the recognition of patients' rights becomes a flight from responsibility. Whether because of fear or because of indifference, overwork, or diffidence, physicians may be prepared to abdicate responsibility for some decisions to patients. Giving patients information, they have discovered, may be easier than withholding it. While a number of observers of the medical scene have argued that patients and patient advocates may demand rights in response to the impersonality of relations with physicians, few have noted that physicians may also become advocates of patients' rights in response to the impersonality of their relations with patients. In this sense, the culture of rights is a product of the very disappearance of the patient. Just as the rise of scientific medicine, an emphasis on technology in diagnosis and treatment, and an indifference to psychological and social factors in disease all imply the absence of interest in the patient as a person, so, too, do they imply the reconstruction of patienthood around a notion of rights.

The culture of rights pervades contemporary medicine, but in intensive care it takes on both an additional significance and a slightly different form. On the one hand, a great deal is at stake in the ICU. On the wards and regular floors, medical decisions are typically routine, at least in the sense that most patients want to be treated and that most physicians want to treat. Although there is no lack of technical complexity, there are fewer points at which physicians or patients are called on to decide whether or not to treat aggressively. In contrast, in the ICU, fundamental decisions about the overall direction of medical care intrude with startling regularity. As a result, one resident told me, keeping patients informed becomes more important, "simply because it is a crisis. . . . Any patient there, by virtue of being there, is in critical condition. . . . They're very much prone to having a deteriorating . . . course, whereas most of the patients in the ward are not like that." In this sense, the culture of rights deepens in response to the very crises that pervade intensive care.

On the other hand, the pace of events is often much faster in the ICU than on wards or on regular floors. This frantic pace, combined with the density of intervention characteristic of the ICU, creates a temptation to go ahead with procedures in the absence of even the formalities, let alone the substance, of consent. As one resident explained, when a patient is deteriorating rapidly, informed consent suffers a little bit just because of necessity of time. Doing a life-saving procedure, one wouldn't go through the elaborate explanation of what it means to put a Swan-Ganz catheter into the right side of the heart, into the pulmonary artery, that you would do if you were, say, on the floor and the patient is about to have a cardiac catheterization, which involves almost the same procedure, . . . basically the same complications, the same risks. It takes, I think, a good cardiologist about fifteen minutes to discuss the procedure and allow the patient to ask questions.

And another observed bluntly: "I don't usually . . . worry about informed consent if I'm trying to save someone's life." Thus, the crisis atmosphere of intensive care reinforces a commitment to rights but also makes that commitment more difficult to realize.

Intensive care also changes the character of that commitment. Most patients in intensive care, as I have taken pains to argue, cannot participate in decisions surrounding their own care by virtue of the very conditions that brought them to the unit. Moreover, it is precisely those patients who are least able to participate for whom general decisions—to intubate or not to intubate, to dialyze or not to dialyze, whether to treat aggressively or unaggressively—are usually most pressing. The result is that the patient's family is typically substituted for the patient himself or herself. "Patients' families," one resident explained, "are often making decisions, more decisions in terms of the patient care. . . . Some of the things that we ordinarily deal through the patient with, we deal with the family."

Thus, to the degree that the patient slips from sight, the family becomes more visible. "Families," according to another resident,

are basically here more than on the wards. They are more aware of the problems. You see them more. On the wards you're all over the hospital and you don't get to see the family every day. Here, usually, you get to see the family every day and so I think they are more informed. Whether or not that's more important, I think that's obvious. It is more important. I think families, people are going to die here and their courses change more quickly here than on the wards.

Indeed, so deeply wedded are the physicians at Outerboro and Countryside to the notion that families should participate in decisions that they will sometimes go to great lengths to create a family, at least for the purposes at hand, even where none exists in a more immediate sense. Consider, for example, the case of Mr. Pike.

Pike, a 59-year-old man who lived alone, had been admitted to Countryside after a cardiac arrest and with a large mass in his lung. Neither his landlord nor any of the few friends who occasionally called the hospital had ever met any of his family, although the landlord did believe that he had once been married and that he may have had a son who he had been out of touch with for many years. In the face of Pike's grim prognosis, John, who was the attending of record in the case, had been prepared to treat unaggressively even in the absence of family. But the prospect made him uncomfortable. On the day of Pike's admission, he had asked if there were any family. When told that there was not, he suggested, "We need to really work on this. Usually there's some family." In the chart, he noted, "I would ask social services to try again to reach his son. Apparently there has been no contact for years." When Ken returned to the unit on the third day of Pike's hospital stay, he was even more cautious. Told of John's willingness to treat Pike unaggressively, he demurred: "This case is different if there are family members around. You can consult with them about his life-style, but this is different." Finally, on the fourth day of Pike's stay, the social service department successfully contacted two daughters. Although neither of the daughters had seen their father for over seven years, Ken agreed to withholding additional support and, eventually, withdrawing support only after he had spoken with them.

My point is not that this is a typical case. It is not. Most patients, particularly at Countryside, have easily identifiable families. My point is only that, in the absence of family, the culture of rights—and, perhaps, the flight from responsibility—is so strong that physicians will go to great lengths to invent one.

In some instances, physicians may develop relationships with families as they have not with patients. One resident, for example, while acknowledging that many of her co-residents did not like talking to families, explained that she did. "In the unit, it's the only kind of personal interaction you have since the patient is completely out of it." Moreover, the ICU physicians at both Outerboro and Countryside often typify families in much the same terms they use for patients. Some they consider difficult or demanding. In a few cases, as with a few patients, they come to feel genuine affection for a father or mother, husband or wife, son or daughter. But the general character of relations with families should not be mistaken. Like relations with patients, according to one resident, it is highly focused:

In the unit the discussions are usually very directed toward three different areas. . . . One is to strictly [apprise] the family of exactly what's wrong and what the care is going to be. The second is to tell them that their family member is dying or has died already. The third, I think, is to address this issue of resuscitation. That usually comes in a period where we think they're dying or we know that they will at some point in the near future or that the disease is utterly irreversible and to treat is to torture. We see the families, I think, almost as much, maybe more, but we're talking about three defined things when we see them in the ICU.

Where, on the floor, physicians may talk to families about long-term plans, in the unit discussions are more usually confined to specific issues.

Thus, the relationship with the family not only substitutes for the relationship with the patient but also comes to mirror it. It is not a personal relationship but one that is functionally specific: the family becomes the carrier of the patients' rights. Thus, the patient is reconstructed. Even lying in a bed comatose and unresponsive, the patient becomes, in a sense, a participant in his or her own medical care. This is not participation in the sense of self-care or self-diagnosis or even in the sense of "cooperating" with a medically prescribed regimen. Neither does it involve control over specific decisions. Indeed, it is not even direct participation, but often substituted participation, when a family acts on behalf of the patient. Rather, it is participation in the sense that decisions are made in the name of the patient's wishes. Thus, the patient is reconstructed, but more or less as an embodiment of will, as an abstraction rather than as a personality.

7

Patients and Families

To say that the intensive care patient has become an abstraction is to adopt the point of view of the doctor and, to some degree, the nurse. Patients—at least those who are awake and alert—do not, of course, think of themselves as abstractions. Neither do husbands or wives, sons or daughters think of their wives and husbands or mothers and fathers as abstractions. We should not be surprised, perhaps, that patients like Naismith Brown (whom I discussed in chapter 3)—themselves potential objects of slights and harsh judgments—welcome the predominantly technical orientation of intensive care and the notion of rights that comes with it. What is surprising, however, is that orientation is also welcomed by patients—and the families of patients—who are, by any account, altogether solid citizens.

To be sure, patients and families alike prefer kindness to cruelty, civility to incivility. Just as any full account of nurses' and doctors' relations with patients must include an acknowledgment of many small acts of kindness, so, too, a full account of patients' relations with nurses and doctors must include an acknowledgment of the deep gratitude those small acts inspire. The nurses, in particular, are often singled out by patients and families for their thoughtfulness. One woman, who had lingered alert in the Outerboro unit for nearly a month—and, thus, had come to know the staff better than most—maintained that it was the nurses who had made her stay tolerable. "The nurses, they were all so supportive. They were so kind and everything." One nurse in particular

was so sweet. She even went as far as to tell me, ask me, what I wanted her to bring me in the morning for breakfast. I said, "No, I don't want anything, that's okay." She said, "Well, if you want anything, you get the nurses at the desk to call me at home." Yes! They'd call around six; they were usually out there when she'd get up. Let her know whatever I wanted her to bring me.

For families of patients, a few kind words are often enough. Thus, the daughter of a 69-year-old man (hospitalized at Countryside after a stroke

complicated by heart disease) described the kindness of a nurse during her
father's first night in the unit.

That was one horrible night for my father. . . . Wendy, my father's nurse that night,
was terrific. God bless her, because I am sure that she was instrumental in keeping
my father alive. . . . The head nurse came down. They must have told her that I was
sitting in the waiting room. I was sitting in the waiting room in the dark, clenching my
fists, shedding some tears. She put her arm around me. She was marvelous. She was
extremely compassionate. And she tried to explain what was happening. And then she
said, "Would you like to come down now and see your father? You can spend some
time." I held his hand, and I talked to him a little bit. I was teasing him. . . . She
hugged me and said that is what you want to remember.

So, too, patients and families want to be kept informed. Although there is
a great deal of variation in how much patients and families want to know, all
of those I spoke to wanted, at the very least, an explanation of basic procedures and schedules. "They didn't just do things and not explain," one Outerboro patient told me. "'We're going to stick a tube up your nose. Lay down
and shut up.' Not at all." And the husband of a 71-year-old woman, admitted
to the Countryside unit after a heart attack, told me, approvingly,

I feel that they are telling me as much as they can. I feel that because I see her two or
three times a day. . . . I've had to ask a couple of questions, which is normal. Most of
the time they have met me or something. . . . Telling me what they were doing and
what to expect.

By the same token, when patients or families feel they are not treated with
respect or not kept informed, they often become angry. Thus, the two sons
of Albert DeLuca, a 60-year-old man with incurable heart disease, told me
with mounting fury of their long wait for news about their father. "Nobody
really tells you what is going on. You can only go under the assumption that
no news is good news for so long before it starts to eat at you. You want
somebody to come out and tell you what the hell is going on." When I suggested that they could call their father's private physician or look for one of
the interns or residents, the older son disagreed:

In a situation like this where, in an intensive care unit, where life is hanging on an
edge, that whoever that person is, should be looking for me. I shouldn't have to be
looking for him, wondering what kind of status my father is. He should be calling me
on the telephone. We would like to speak with the DeLuca family or whatever. Let us
know what is going on rather than us having to sit and wonder.

Along with his brother and mother, he continued, he had, on the advice some
days earlier of his father's physicians, alerted a wide network of relatives that
his father's situation was critical. Now that he had heard from a nurse that

his father was scheduled to leave the unit, his relief was matched by confusion and embarrassment:

And we have gone from a situation where they said, "Don't leave the hospital," to now where he is coming out of intensive care. Does that mean that we can call our relatives and tell them they don't have to fly here from all across the country because he is going to be okay? The fact that they are taking him out of intensive care, does that mean that he is getting better or that he is just not as sick as he was so they are going to give the room to somebody else? What is it? We don't know that.

But none of this is remarkable. To say that patients and families prefer to be treated with kindness or that they want basic information is not to say that they want a deep or personal relationship with doctors and nurses. Indeed, some of the high praise for nurses comes precisely from the recognition, as the daughter of one patient put it, that they are "taking care of this person that you love so much, who they obviously don't know from Adam." Preferring kindness or wanting information represents a level of expectation no higher than that attached to a repairman or technician—albeit in circumstances far more charged emotionally. What is remarkable is not how much personal attention patients and families expect from physicians and nurses, but how little.

For patients and families alike, a transfer to intensive care is a frightening experience. "I got scared," Tom Connors told me about his initial reaction when his daughter, Kelly, was taken to the Countryside unit, "because only very, very sick people go on respirators." But what is frightening is not so much the unit as the brute facts of acute illness. If anything, the unit, as distinct from the illness that requires transfer to it, is reassuring. At first, the wife of a man with cirrhosis of the liver told me, she had been scared: "All the stuff was on him. The constant attention scared me at first. As far as their being there, right at the desk in front, that to me means watch and alert." But, she continued, she soon realized that the very equipment and the constant attention that at first frightened her could also be a source of comfort: "Then after a while I got comfortable with that. Now I am glad that they watch everything. If something changes, they jump. They are fast. They don't fool around." A man who had been intubated at Outerboro made a similar observation, even more graphically:

A lot of doctors and nurses, and they put into your mouth and lungs, you know. I don't know, just some kind of thing about that. And I cry because, you know, those people are on top of you and you don't . . . and you feel it, too, and they're trying to put it in your stomach . . . for breath, because that machine they want to help me to breathe because I cannot breathe by myself. . . . It's a good feeling because all those doctors are taking care of you, you know. They're fighting for your life. They don't know you, but they're there fighting for your life. . . . I was scared because . . . I don't know what is going to happen. But I was relieved because the doctors, those people, are on top of you anytime. You feel like scared but safe. It's incredible.

In the face of acute, often life-threatening illness, neither patients nor families are concerned primarily with civility or kindness. They want the illness treated, the crisis managed. It matters more that the nurses are available than that they are pleasant, more that the doctors are competent than that they are personable. And the enormous technical apparatus of intensive care seems less intimidating than a potential source of life. "I was totally amazed," Mrs. Franco, the wife of one patient, told me,

at all they give him. Like one day they want to bring his blood pressure up and the next day they want to bring it down. They can do it so easily. And seeing where they put in these central lines is fantastic. Because when he went downstairs [out of the unit] and they had to draw blood, that nurse couldn't even get blood from him.

"Happiness, unhappiness, none of that played a part in it," Lee Donald told me as he was recovering from an episode of acute renal failure.

The thing that I was concerned about was that I had almost died and intervention stopped that. I was pleased with that. They kept me alive. I wasn't unhappy. There was no reason to be unhappy. I wasn't there long enough to make any kind of judgment about happiness, unhappiness, like and dislike. The things that were done needed to be done. . . . It was your life that you were trying to fix up. That's all that I can say.

If, at times, technology appears to be a substitute for a more personal touch, this seems to most patients and families an altogether acceptable trade-off.

The willingness of patients and families to trade personal relationships for technical competence is particularly apparent in their stance toward private family physicians. Although many of the unit patients and their families felt deep affection for and placed considerable trust in private physicians, most of the patients and *all* of the families I talked to were prepared to distinguish intensive care from other circumstances.[1] Edwin Landreaux, for ex-

---

1. One of the exceptions is instructive. Carol Regan was bitter over her care in the unit and repeated insistently over the course of my interview with her that her regular physician—who had treated her for many years for her chronic renal failure—would have handled matters differently. But Regan, unlike the majority of ICU patients, was not in a life-threatening situation. Moreover, Regan was on methadone maintenance and had been denied her methadone in the unit until her regular physician's secretary intervened on her behalf. "They weren't giving me my meds," she told me insistently. Regan was not a "solid citizen" distressed by the impersonality of intensive care but (at least briefly) an object of reform distressed that the unit's orientation was too personal.

ample, told me that he and his wife had been "very happy" with a doctor they had known for over a decade. But he did not see any need for that physician to follow his wife in intensive care: "Not saying anything against our family doctor, but I think they are probably better informed as far as hearts are concerned. This is the main issue." Similarly, Alberto Rodriguez told me that it was, in general, better to have a doctor "who knows you well, who you see lots of times." But in intensive care, "you know you are fighting for your life. When you see all those different doctors, you start thinking, they are taking good care of me. . . . But when you are out there and then come over here [to a ward bed], then you want one doctor."

While the kindness of nurses and doctors is appreciated, none of the patients or families I talked to confused that kindness with the more important emotional support they received from additional family and friends. In fact, many families, in particular, found the very notion of doctors and nurses offering emotional support a discomfiting one:

I don't think they should. . . . Doctors and nurses probably shouldn't be emotional with their patients. The way I understood it from years and years back, they are there to do a job and not to be emotional. They are trained for that.

I know that there are certain people that are very empathetic to what you are experiencing but . . . it's hard. They care for a lot of people. So it's real hard for them when they are taking care of the patients also [to] be able to really and truly support the family. They can't. They can't leave the patient to go out and let you cry on their shoulder. . . . They do a good job, letting you know that they are there and that they care. But I don't think you can really share too much with them.

Indeed, many patients and families neither knew nor even cared to know the names of the doctors and nurses who had seen them through the unit. Two weeks after his daughter had first been brought to Countryside, Tom Connors had learned to read the monitors that recorded Kelly's heart beat and respiration. He could tell me about the drugs Kelly was receiving. But when I asked him if he could remember the names of the doctors who had first treated Kelly, he told me he could not. I asked him if he knew the names of the doctors treating her at the time we talked. He told me that he did not: "If you don't have a name that is tough to pronounce, you don't get into doctor school. I don't care about names as long as I can recognize you and know that you are working with my kid." There was no lack of emotion in Tom Connors's account of his daughter's hospitalization—but it was emotion focused on his daughter's illness, not on the doctors and nurses who were treating her.

Still, there is also a warning in Tom Connors's comments. Although he neither knew nor cared to know the names of the physicians caring for his daughter, "If I have a question, I'm going to nail you." In return for tolerating a certain impersonality of care, Tom expected not only a high quality of technical care but also the right to make key decisions bearing on his daughter's care. Few of the patients I talked to (all of whom, recall, had been awake and alert throughout their ICU stay) claimed to have participated in key decisions nor, in many cases, could they even identify a key decision. Neither could the families of patients whose course in the unit had been both brief and successful. However, the situation was very different among families of patients in more critical condition. These families simply assumed that key decisions would be theirs.

When, for example, I asked the older of Mr. DeLuca's sons what he would do if his father's condition deteriorated, he acknowledged that it was a difficult question.

I don't know. Sometimes I think, if it was just the machine and he needed the machine to stay alive, if it were me, maybe shut it off. But with my father, he has been in this situation two or three times now. Each time they've written him off and he's come back. . . . I don't know what I'd do in a situation like that. If I was absolutely convinced that there was no way he could come out of it, then I'd probably tell them to shut the machine off. But I'd have to be 100 percent. If there was just a shadow of doubt, I'd hang in there. . . . If they weren't capable of making the decision then, if there was any doubt in my mind, I'd leave it on until everything was exhausted.

Thus, Edward DeLuca was prepared to weigh his father's history against his own preferences. He understood the gravity of the choice. But no physician appeared in his account of how he would decide. If he were convinced that his father could not recover, he would *tell* them to shut the machine off.

If families believe that decisions are theirs, it is at least in part because physicians have told them so. June Russell, for example, explained that, when her mother's surgeon proposed amputating her mother's leg, "I was told that I would be asked to sign something."

Of course, then we thought that death was imminent, like maybe an hour away. Then I consulted with my family. I was the oldest child, and I was the only child that was here at that moment. And I said what should we do? If Mom is going to pass away anyway, should we take this leg off? Do we want to think of her like that, or what do we want to do? Help me, because I know I am the one that has to sign.

Eventually Mrs. Russell agreed to the amputation, after consulting with another physician who had been treating her mother for a chronic condition. But even though she allowed herself to be convinced, she still thought of the ultimate decision as her own: "We were really almost not going to sign the permit."

The sense of empowerment I found among many of the families is a product of the culture of rights. Yet it also contains the potential for conflict. Physicians are prepared to empower families in the broad direction of medical care—to decide whether to treat aggressively or unaggressively. They are not prepared, however, to empower families to make specific decisions, decisions that they see as falling within the proper realm of technique. But families are not always prepared to make this fine distinction. Mrs. Franco, for example, acknowledged that the physicians had honored her wishes when "I didn't want anything cut, anything taken away from him." Moreover, she assumed that she would be consulted about any decision to discontinue her husband's respirator. However, she had also been upset when her husband had been transferred briefly out of the Intensive Care Unit soon after his severe stroke. She had spoken with John, the unit's director: "I asked him if the family would be called in on the decisions. And he says we will be made aware of what's going on. So I don't think we actually have, like I haven't had any decision making at all."

For the most part, then, there is a happy fit between the expectations of doctors and nurses, on one hand, and the expectations of patients and their families, on the other. Doctors and nurses have little interest in the patient as a person. Patients expect from physicians and nurses technical expertise and little more. Physicians and nurses are prepared to acknowledge the rights of patients. Families are prepared to claim those rights on behalf of patients. It is around these mutual expectations that patienthood is reconstructed in the ICU.

But all is not so simple. The culture of rights also creates its own tensions. If physicians are prepared to acknowledge the rights of patients in the broad direction of medical care, they are also insistent on reserving some decisions to themselves as matters of technique. Families do not always agree. Thus, the lines of conflict are drawn. The point in question is not whether patients have rights. All agree that they do. Neither is the question whether those rights may be exercised on behalf of the patient by the patient's family. Most agree that they may. Rather, the issue becomes one of the limits of rights, of the boundaries between matters of value and matters of technical knowledge. It is to these issues that I turn in part II.

Part 2

MEDICAL ETHICS: TRIAGE AND
THE LIMITATION OF TREATMENT

Among the doctors and nurses who work in the intensive care units at Outerboro and Countryside hospitals, one concern dominates all others. It is a concern raised almost daily during rounds, repeated endlessly in casual conversation, reiterated with insistent regularity in interviews. It is a concern both deeply personal and highly principled. The intensive care unit is filled with too many patients dying long and agonizing deaths, beyond the help of medicine, filling beds better used by those with some more reasonable chance of recovery. "My big thing is quality of life," one Countryside intern told me.

I wouldn't want to see my parents in a situation here in the unit. I myself wouldn't like to be in the unit. I wouldn't want to be brain-dead on a ventilator. Some of our patents are close to being brain-dead. . . . Mr. K. is one. He's got zero quality of life. He's got zero cure.

At Outerboro, the concern is even more intense. "There are frustrations," one resident there explained, "taking care of a lot of people who you just don't think belong there at all."

They should never have been admitted to the unit because they have an end stage disease and the chances of recovery are nil. And those are the ones who actually stay in the beds the longest period of time because they don't die quickly, because we can't kill them. So that I find very frustrating. Each time through the ICU is a little bit different. There's a different flavor, and sometimes you'll come in and 90 percent of the beds are brain-dead people. It's very depressing. It's a terrible use of ICU beds.

This is a powerful concern but also an unsettling one. On the one hand, it is reassuring to find physicians and nurses frustrated by their inability to help patients. It is a frustration born of their very commitment to healing. On the other hand, it is far from reassuring to find doctors and nurses who, unable

99

to heal patients, are then prepared to abandon those patients, complaining only—in stark, and perhaps overdramatic, language—that "we can't kill them." Moreover, it is unsettling to encounter in physicians and nurses, those to whom we look to master illness, so overwhelming a sense of impotence. The very women and men who run intensive care units seem unable to control them. Not only does death continue to defy them, but so too do the very tools produced to forestall death. Underlying the concern that the ICU is treating too many dying patients is an image of medicine out of control—doctors and nurses unable to stop treatment when treatment no longer has a purpose, unable to turn their considerable skills to the advantage of those who need them most.

The doctors' and nurses' concern that intensive care units are treating too many terminally ill patients and treating them for too long expresses two of the central issues in contemporary medical ethics. First, it expresses issues about the ways in which resources are allocated. If there are only a limited number of beds in an intensive care unit, who should use those beds, how should the decision be made, by whom, and by what criteria? I return to these issues in chapter 14. Second, it expresses issues about the limitation of treatment. Under what circumstances, if any, is it acceptable to withhold or withdraw treatments that might extend the life of a patient? How should that decision be made, by whom, and by what criteria? To these questions I turn more immediately.

Questions surrounding the limitation of treatment have generated rich literatures in medical ethics, filled with fine distinctions and carefully drawn conclusions from clearly formulated principles. But medical ethics is one thing; medical practice is quite another. This chapter and the succeeding ones are not about ethics in a conventional sense—about what is right and wrong, what is permissible and what not. They are not about how decisions should be made but about how they are in fact made.

Most generally (and to borrow a phrase), physicians make decisions, but not under conditions of their own choosing. It is, to be sure, the physician who writes the final order to continue or discontinue dialysis, to transfuse blood, to turn off a respirator. But ethicists, the courts, and, increasingly, legislatures have also specified some of the circumstances in which they consider limitation of treatment permissible and some of the circumstances in which they do not. Administrators, worried about finances, legal liabilities, and any number of other matters, set hospital policy. Nurses may have views of their own, and those views are not always the same as physicians'. And, most important, patients or—in the frequent circumstances in which dying patients are unable to do so for themselves—patients' families press their wishes with greater or lesser insistence. From the sociologist's point of view, much of the drama of intensive care comes from the efforts of physicians to maintain their discretion in decisions bearing on nothing less than matters of life and death.[1]

To physicians, discretion may be an end in itself. But it is not *only* an end in itself. In particular, physicians most often use their discretion—albeit with occasional exceptions—to limit treatment. This is, in itself, a major finding of the research reported here. The impression that emerges from some of the most publicized cases of termination of treatment is, of course, somewhat different. The landmark Quinlan case in New Jersey, the ruling by the United States Supreme Court in the Cruzan case, and a long list of so-called Baby Doe cases all involved families, not physicians, suing to have treatment terminated. Yet these cases are deceptive. They represent special situations in that the objection to terminating treatment was raised neither by family nor by physicians but by hospital administrators (the Quinlan case), a state government (the Cruzan case), or the federal government (the Baby Doe cases). Each was a test case, far removed from the usual practice of medical decision making. Moreover, they reflect physicians' limited standing, on these issues, in courts of law. Physicians, unlike families, are ill-equipped to sue for termination of treatment. Nonetheless, in practice, if not in law, physicians do exert considerable influence. "It's rarely the family themselves," one Outerboro resident told me, "who come forward and say, 'We want nothing more done.'" As a result, whatever happens later, it is almost always physicians—"80 or 90 percent of the time," according to one Countryside intern—who initiate discussions about limiting treatment. Moreover, as we will see in considerable detail later, when there is conflict over limitation of treatment, it is typically between physicians prepared to limit their efforts and families asking them to "do everything."[2]

1. My choice of the term "discretion" rather than the perhaps more conventional term, "authority," is altogether intentional. It is precisely my point that physicians are able to maintain discretion—an ability to do more or less as they like—only by abandoning authority with the tightly linked claim that they have a *right* to make decisions.

2. For evidence that physicians are more inclined to limit treatment than are patients or their families, see Marion Danis, Sandra J. Jarr, Leslie I. Southerland, Rosemary Nocella, and Donald L. Patrick, "A Comparison of Patient, Family, and Nurse Evaluations of the Usefulness of Intensive Care," *Critical Care Medicine* 15 (1987): 138–43; Marion Danis, Martha Susan Gerrity, Leslie Irene Southerland, and Donald Lee Patrick, "A Comparison of Patient, Family, and

By long tradition, physicians put practice before theory. They are not ac-customed to justifying their decisions in any terms but medical ones or to articulating general principles.[3] But the rise of medical ethics as a social movement, along with the development of a culture of rights, has changed all that. In the face of patients' rights and the sometimes abstract distinctions favored by ethicists and lawyers, physicians must not only justify themselves but do so in terms that at the very least take general principles into account. Physicians, whether they want to or not, have entered the realm of ideology.

In defending their discretion against families—as well as against courts, ethicists, hospital administrators, and other challengers—physicians have developed a number of distinctive strategies. First, physicians do not typi-cally defend their discretion by claiming explicit jurisdiction over matters of ethics and values. Rather, when physicians do resist the wishes of patients and their families, at both Outerboro and Countryside, they justify that re-sistance by moving decisions from the realm of values to the realm of tech-nique. Indeed, physicians rarely question the values of their patients. To the contrary, physicians typically assume a stance of strict value neutrality. How-ever, at the same time, they argue, frequently and insistently, that some de-cisions are not value laden at all but simply technical. As such, physicians would argue, they are beyond the proper range not only of patients and fam-ilies but of both the law and ethics. The physician's defense of discretion, then, is an effort, characteristic of American professions more generally, to convert expertise to the legitimation of authority.[4]

Second, much of what appears to be a decision about limitation of treat-ment is often better understood as the representation or dramatization of a decision. Few decisions to limit treatment are discrete events. They are, rather, the result of an incremental process consisting of many smaller deci-sions that often sneak up, almost imperceptibly, on doctors and patients alike. Yet medical ethics and the law have joined in insisting that physicians present decisions as if they were discrete. Doctors have complied, especially in the ways in which they document their decisions. Written orders not to

Physician Assessments of the Value of Medical Intensive Care," *Critical Care Medicine* 16 (1988): 594–600; Marion Danis, Donald L. Patrick, Leslie I. Southerland, and Michael L. Green, "Patients' and Families' Prefences for Medical Intensive Care," *Journal of the American Medical Association* 260 (1988): 797–802.

3. I am indebted to an anonymous reviewer for the University of Chicago Press for this formulation.

4. See, for example, Magali Sarfatti Larson, *The Rise of Professionalism* (Berkeley: University of California Press, 1977); Eliot Freidson, *Professional Powers* (Chicago: University of Chicago Press, 1986).

resuscitate a patient, at Outerboro in particular, often take on the character of a public performance. On the one hand, it is important to see through that performance to the "real" process of decision making. On the other hand, the performance itself takes on a symbolic significance important in its own right.

The agenda ahead is, then, a complex one. Chapter 8, organized around the concept of "torture" as it is used at both Countryside and Outerboro, discusses the reasons physicians and nurses want to limit treatment. Chapter 9, organized around the concept of "uncertainty," describes how physicians, acting collectively, impose an obligation to treat on themselves that goes beyond what most, acting individually, would want. Chapter 10 examines the way physicians use the concepts of the "terminal patient" and "aggressive treatment" to restore some degree of discretion in the face of threats to it. Finally, chapters 11 through 13 examine physicians' responses to families and the law.

8

"Penguins in the Basement"

At the Outerboro ICU, physicians limited at least some form of potentially life-prolonging treatment for roughly one in seven patients. At Countryside, unit physicians limited at least some form of potentially life-prolonging treatment for roughly one in four. Decisions to limit treatment play a prominent part in intensive care units. But decisions to continue treatment play an even more prominent part in the imagination of the doctors and nurses who work in those units. At Countryside, some of the attending physicians, most of the housestaff, and nearly all of the nursing staff are stridently critical of the unit for treating patients too aggressively. An intern:

> I think patients who have end stage disease, who are in [their] seventies or eighties, should not be intubated and brought to the unit under any circumstance. I kind of have an aggressive attitude as far as what some people might call euthanasia. I think that there are cancer patients that are there that have no prognosis and the same with AIDS patients. . . . [They are] either going to die now or go to the ICU for two weeks and be tortured with needles and procedures [and then die].

At Outerboro, the criticism is even more frequent and more strident. A nurse, in excruciating detail:

> I've been mad lately because we've gotten a lot of young people who are brain-dead, with drug overdoses, stuff like that. They let these patients linger in these beds. I've actually seen patients rot in a bed. It drives me crazy that someone doesn't make the decision. . . . Just have a little balls and take the person off the ventilator, because you're not going to save their lives. . . . We have one guy who had no blood flow from the neck up, so his brain was gone. He stayed in that bed for two and a half months with a heart beat. . . . We were watching things fall off. Fingernails were falling off.

Nearly two-thirds of the patients admitted to the intensive care units at both Outerboro and Countryside eventually leave the hospital alive. Yet the ICU resident I cited in the introduction to part II was prepared to claim that "sometimes . . . 90 percent of the beds are brain-dead people." The claim is an exaggeration. As a statement about the distribution of patients, it is easily dismissed. But as a statement about the felt reality of intensive care medicine, it requires explanation.

Limiting Treatment

How often do physicians limit potentially life-prolonging treatment for ICU patients? The unit physicians at Outerboro explicitly discussed limiting treatment for 57 (24 percent) of 233 patients who were discharged from or died in the unit. They in fact limited some form of treatment for 35 (15 percent) (see fig. 8.1). At Countryside, unit physicians limited treatment even more frequently. There, the unit physicians discussed limiting treatment for 39 (33 percent) of 117 deaths and discharges. They in fact limited treatment for 32 (27 percent) (see fig. 8.2). Although directly comparable data from other hospitals are hard to come by, it would seem that Outerboro tends toward the low end among American hospitals in the frequency with which physicians limit treatment while Countryside falls more clearly at the high end.[1]

1. Most other research on the "epidemiology" of treatment limitation is based on chart reviews rather than direct observation of the decision-making process. It has, consequently, focused on Do Not Resuscitate orders, relatively well documented in charts, rather than on the limitation of treatment more generally. Moreover, in making sense of reported distributions of DNR orders, it is essential to keep in mind differences in severity of illness. In any event, one study of three Texas teaching hospitals found that 9 percent of a sample of 758 patients had been made DNR and another 10 percent had been seriously discussed for such an order. Andrew L. Evans and Baruch A. Brody, "The Do Not Resuscitate Order in Teaching Hospitals," *Journal of the American Medical Association* 253 (1985): 2236–39. A similar study of three California teaching hospitals found that DNR orders were considered for 4 percent and eventually written for 3 percent of a sample of 3,000 admissions. Bernard Lo, Glenn Saika, William Strull, Elizabeth Thomas, and Jonathan Showstack, "'Do Not Resuscitate' Decisions: A Prospective Study at Three Teaching Hospitals," *Archives of Internal Medicine* 145 (1985): 115–17. A 1980 study of the Portland Veterans Administration Medical Center and a 1984 study of New York Hospital also found that DNR orders were issued for approximately 3 percent of admissions. Richard Uhlmann, Walter McDonald, and Thomas Inui, "Epidemiology of No-Code Orders in an Academic Hospital," *Western Journal of Medicine* 140 (1984): 114–16; Mary E. Charlson, Frederic L. Sax, Ronald MacKenzie, Suzanne D. Fields, Robert L. Braham, and R. Gordon Douglas, Jr., "Resuscitation: How Do We Decide?" *Journal of the American Medical Association* 255 (1986): 1316–22. A study of a community hospital in the San Francisco Bay area found that the 333 patients for whom DNR orders had been issued over a six-month period constituted only 3 percent of discharges but fully 70 percent of all patients who died in the hospital during that time. Helene Levens Lipton, "Do-Not-Resuscitate Decisions in a Community Hospital," *Journal of the American Medical Association* 256 (1986): 1164–69. Similarly, a study of a university-affiliated teaching hospital found that DNR orders were written for 68 percent of patients who died in-hospital over three-month periods in 1982 and 1986. Palmi V. Jonsson, Michael McNamee, and Edward W. Campion, "The 'Do Not Resuscitate' Order: A Profile of Its Chang-

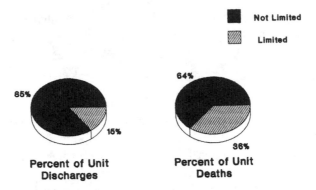

Figure 8.1. The limitation of treatment, Outerboro.

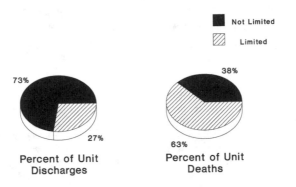

Figure 8.2. The limitation of treatment, Countryside.

ing Use," *Archives of Internal Medicine* 148 (1988): 2373–75. In a somewhat more specialized study—and one more directly comparable to the research reported here—of 506 admissions to the ten-bed MICU of University Hospitals of Cleveland, DNR orders were issued in 71 (14 percent) of the cases. Stewart J. Youngner, Wendy Lewandowski, Donna K. McLish, Barbara W. Juknialis, Claudia Coulton, and Edward T. Bartlett, "'Do Not Resuscitate' Orders: Incidence and Implications in a Medical Intensive Care Unit," *Journal of the American Medical Association* 253 (1985): 54–57. In the most ambitious study of the epidemiology of DNR orders, a study of more than 7,000 admissions in the ICUs of thirteen different hospitals, the George Washington University ICU Research Unit found that DNR orders were issued in 6.2 percent of all cases and accounted for 39 percent of all ICU deaths. Jack E. Zimmerman, William A. Knaus, Steven M. Sharpe, Andrew S. Anderson, Elizabeth Draper, and Douglas Wagner, "The Use and Implications of Do Not Resuscitate Orders in Intensive Care Units," *Journal of the American Medical Association* 255 (1986): 351–56. Finally, a study of 1,719 patients admitted to the intensive care units at Moffit-Long University Hospital in San Francisco and the San Francisco General Hospital showed that life support—a somehat broader category than DNR orders—was withheld from 1 percent and withdrawn from 5 percent of patients, accounting for 45 percent of unit deaths. Nicholas G. Smerda, Bradley H. Evans, Linda S. Grais, Neal H. Cohen, Bernard Lo,

If we limit our count to those patients who died without leaving the hospital—in effect, a broad definition of dying patients—the proportions are even higher. At Outerboro, the unit physicians limited treatment for 33 (36 percent) of 92 such patients. At Countryside, they limited treatment for no less than 25 (63 percent) of 40. From this perspective, the limitation of treatment would seem common practice in both units. Physicians at Outerboro limit treatment for a substantial minority of dying patients. Physicians at Countryside limit treatment for a majority of such patients. Yet this is not how physicians and nurses experience the unit.

First, virtually all patients are treated actively in the intensive care unit at least at the time of their admission. American medicine, in general, is committed to active treatment, and the ICU is simply the site in which that commitment is played out. "I think it has to do with the concept of what medicine is," one Outerboro resident suggested, "that we believe in the cure, and we look at death as the enemy and we are gladiators in the battle against disease. . . . You send a patient to the ICU to escalate the battle, so this is the next logical step in that battle." To be sure, an occasional patient is admitted to the units at both Outerboro and Countryside for intensive nursing care with the stipulation that he or she is not to be resuscitated in the event of a cardiac arrest or not to be placed on a respirator. For the most part, however, if a patient and physician have agreed in advance that the patient is not to be resuscitated or not to be placed on a respirator, that patient is considerably less likely to find a place in the unit to begin with. Because intensive care units are densely staffed with nurses and physicians and equipped with sophisticated equipment, it makes little sense to admit patients unless there is some intention to use those very substantial resources. In this sense, active treatment, at least at the time of admission, emerges out of the very mission of intensive care.

Second, decisions to limit treatment typically come only after a patient has been admitted to the unit. More often than not, this decision comes only at the end of a patient's stay in the unit, often followed quickly by either death or discharge. The thirty-five patients for whom treatment was limited at Outerboro were in the unit for a cumulative total of 305 days before a decision to limit any treatment was made. They remained in the unit a cumulative total of only 146 days after that decision. Thirty-two patients at Coun-

Molly Cooke, William P. Schecter, Carol Fink, Eve Epstein Jaffe, Christine May, and John M. Luce, "Withholding and Withdrawal of Life Support from the Critically Ill," *New England Journal of Medicine* 322 (1990): 309–15.

tryside were in the unit for a cumulative total of 92 days before a decision was made to limit any treatment. They remained in the unit a cumulative total of only 48 days after that decision. Although, in the end, intensive care physicians limit some form of treatment for a substantial proportion of dying patients, that end does not always come quickly.

Third, limiting some form of potentially life-prolonging treatment is not equivalent to limiting all forms of treatment. The Outerboro physicians never terminate all forms of potentially life-prolonging treatment; the Countryside physicians, only occasionally. More often, they decide to limit step by step. The single most frequent decision to limit treatment is the "Do Not Resuscitate" (DNR) order—written in twenty-five cases at Outerboro and thirty at Countryside.[2] But the DNR order involves nothing more than a contingency. It is a decision not to attempt cardiopulmonary resuscitation *in the event* of a cardiac or respiratory arrest. Thus, a DNR order does not necessarily imply a reduction of therapeutic efforts other than in regard to cardiopulmonary resuscitation in particular. As one Outerboro attending explained,

DNR means what it means. It means do not resuscitate. So, if a lightning bolt hits him and he dies, you don't resuscitate him. That's all it means. It doesn't mean that you don't give whatever support is appropriate to maintain life. They are two very separate issues.

To be sure, in some cases, the Do Not Resuscitate order is accompanied by a general reduction of therapeutic efforts. In others, however, a DNR order is accompanied by what is, in the language of sports and games frequent to medical practice, a "full court press." Beyond writing DNR orders, the Outerboro and Countryside physicians also withheld, in one or more cases, intubation and ventilator support (from patients in respiratory distress), dialysis (from patients with kidney disease), vasopressors (a group of drugs used to manage blood pressure), blood transfusions, antibiotics, and a variety of diagnostic procedures (ranging from taking X-rays and blood samples to the insertion of lines used to monitor cardiac output). But in these instances, too, the decision to limit a particular treatment may be made either alone or in conjunction with other such decisions.

Fourth, a decision to withhold some future treatment—whether cardiopulmonary resuscitation or dialysis—does not imply a decision to withdraw treatments already begun. Indeed, at Outerboro, although physicians did, on

2. For a general discussion of DNR orders, see Stuart J. Youngner, "Do-Not-Resuscitate Orders: No Longer Secret, but Still a Problem," *Hastings Center Report* 17 (1987): 24–33.

occasion, withhold respirator care, they never, in the course of my research, withdrew that care once begun from a respirator-dependent patient. Thus, in one case at Outerboro, a patient remained on a respirator in the unit for eighteen days after he had been made DNR. In another, a patient remained on a respirator in the unit for twenty-six days after a decision not to dialyze despite her kidney failure. (I will have more to say later about the implications of the distinction between withholding and withdrawing treatment.) Countryside, however, is different. There physicians both withhold and withdraw respirator care. In twelve cases they performed a procedure called, in only mildly obscurantist language, a "terminal wean." (Although neither doctors nor nurses literally "pull the plug," the process is dramatic enough. After a doctor or, more often, a nurse turns down the respirator setting, death usually follows quickly, most often in an hour or two.) These twelve cases constitute the only cases at either hospital in which physicians, in effect, stopped all potentially life-prolonging treatments.

From one perspective, then, the physicians at Outerboro and (even more so) Countryside limit treatment frequently—for between one-seventh and one-quarter of all patients they discharge, for between a third and two-thirds of dying patients. But this is not how doctors and nurses experience intensive care. From their point of view, at any given time, they are treating a majority of patients, even those they believe to be incurable. And when they do limit treatment, they do so only partially and then toward the end of the patient's ICU stay. If the doctors and nurses who work in intensive care units are looking for cases of active treatment, they do not have to look far or hard.

Torture

Physicians are, by and large, a compulsive lot. By both training and, perhaps, personality, they are inclined toward activism. In searching for a diagnosis, in searching for a treatment, they are prepared to look beneath each stone, behind each tree. (One of the most frequently repeated aphorisms of medical school advises medical students and housestaff, "When you hear hoofbeats, look for a zebra." Extra credit accrues to the student or young house officer who makes an unusual diagnosis.) In intensive care, where the ability to make a diagnosis or identify the right treatment is often genuinely a matter of life or death, compulsiveness is redoubled. "I don't know what it is," one Outerboro resident told me:

It seems to be, when you bring enough doctors together, [there's] a fear of not doing enough in other people's eyes. . . . Like Mr. Daniels. We gave up on him for dead,

[and] one of the residents said, "Maybe he's getting better. Let's draw blood." So the whole thing started again. . . . I had trouble giving up on Mr. Brown. . . . I just relate to him. . . . I was the one on rounds that, I said, "Maybe we should put a Swan in." I couldn't believe I was saying it.

At the same time, physicians like to think that they are compassionate. If they cannot always cure, they can at least minimize pain. Certainly, physicians do not like to think that they are a source of suffering. Perhaps the most famous maxim in the long history of medical ethics enjoins them, "Above all, do no harm." In most circumstances, the compulsiveness of physicians and their compassion coexist in an easy harmony. Indeed, compulsiveness is the very cornerstone of good treatment. This is as true in intensive care as in any other medical setting. Yet in intensive care the insistent presence of incurably ill patients subtly transforms the relationship between compulsiveness and the injunction to do no harm, between the potential for cure and the intensity of pain.

On the one hand, the compulsive search for a diagnosis or the willingness to try one last treatment may involve procedures that are painful for a patient. If there is a chance of recovery, that pain is justified easily enough. It is less easily justified in an incurable patient. Moreover, among incurable patients, some treatments may simply extend a life that is already wracked by suffering. On the other hand, a willingness to withhold treatment in the name of compassion requires a renunciation of the compulsive search for cure. The incurable patient creates tensions that resonate at the very core of the physician's occupational identity.

These tensions are not ones that physicians resolve easily. An Outerboro intern still struggling to adapt to the demands of medical practice told me the following dream, which includes the image from which the title of this chapter is drawn. He had been invited for dinner by one of the attending physicians, an oncologist. He was in the attending's house

in his basement. And I walk down there and [there were] these penguins in his basements and they were sort of sitting on this table. There was ice scattered around, clearly like the ice was supposed to be there to make them more comfortable so they could live in the proper habitat. But the ice was sort of sitting on the table and melting, and . . . it was just a matter of time until they died. . . . There was also a blender on the table. So I put one of the penguins into the blender and took a whole bunch of ice and put it in the blender as well, because by mixing them all up in the cold circumstance I could presumably prolong their life. I turned on the blender and spun the penguin around and then stopped the blender. And I had apparently succeeded in what I was trying to do, because he was now in a very cold environment. But he was in a pool of blood. Then I woke up.

To make sense of this dream requires neither in-depth analysis nor dubious explorations of a Freudian unconscious. It is a simple statement. In the very effort to treat, the cure may be worse than the disease.

A similar notion recurs in a term that is part of the folklore of the Outerboro ICU, "cheechee." The origin of the term is a joke that was repeated to me on a number of occasions. Like many jokes of its sort, it is not particularly funny and the skill of its telling is in the ability to draw it out in gruesome detail. In one of the briefer versions:

Missionaries are in a tribal land and are captured by the natives. They're brought before the chief and the chief asks one of the missionaries, "What would you prefer, cheechee or death?" And the first missionary says cheechee, at which point the entire tribe descends on him, ties him to a pole. Each member of the tribe [beats] him. And then the rope [is] tied around his hands, and he's dragged about a mile losing bits and pieces of himself. And [he's] thrown over into a ravine. The other missionary looks horrified at what is going on. And the chief comes back to him and asks him, "Well, what do you prefer, death or cheechee?" The missionary looks horrified and thinks, and then says, "I never thought I'd say this, but I would prefer death." The chieftain says, "Yes, but first a little cheechee."

The joke is a precise metaphor. Death is certain. (In most versions of the joke, it is explicit that the first missionary dies from the beatings.) What appears to be a choice is really no choice at all. But death cannot come quickly. In the joke, it must be preceded by "cheechee." In the ICU, it must be preceded by treatment.

"Cheechee" is used by both doctors and nurses at Outerboro almost interchangeably with the word "torture." Both cheechee and torture refer primarily to the extensive treatment of patients who are apparently incurable. (The only instance in which I heard a doctor use either term in relation to a patient who ultimately survived the unit was in reference to a woman whose medical problems were blatantly iatrogenic.) Two Outerboro residents explained:

I think that cheechee is doing all sorts of painful and abusive things to somebody in an attempt to make a diagnosis or perform a therapy. Frequently, we will do that to people who will die no matter what we do.

What I mean by torture is, when you think someone has no reasonable prognosis of getting back to a reasonable life-style that they are themselves comfortable with, I think you've gone beyond the point where you should artificially prolong their life. That means by means of a respirator, by means of blood pressure, by means of pressors to maintain their blood pressure, by means of dialysis, by means of antibiotics with recurrent sepsis. I think torture is a word used to say that we are putting someone through pain without reason, without reasonable hope that we can reverse the pain he has. And that's what I mean by torture.

Although the term "cheechee" is used not at all at Countryside and the term "torture" less often, it is used occasionally and in a sense identical to that at Outerboro. For example, one intern was complaining after a particularly difficult night on call that "the privates come in, and everyone thinks his patient is the most important and wants to go over the subtleties of ESRD [end stage renal disease] with you." He added that he had never seen a dialysis patient get better. "They come in and you treat them and they die. There are two torture machines. There's the rack and then there's the dialysis machine."

Torture, as the ICU staff uses the term, involves both inflicting pain and a sense that the treatments which cause pain are ultimately futile. It is, on the surface, a notion at once compassionate and patient-centered. Yet there is also something curious in the notion, for neither the doctors nor the nurses who use the term are at all sure of how much pain their patients are suffering. Pain is a notoriously difficult phenomenon to measure.[3] Certainly, pain does not lend itself to the sort of precise measurements that are available for rates of respiration or densities of red blood cells. Pain is all the more difficult to measure in dying patients, many of whom are comatose and unresponsive. To be sure, some patients, even those who are otherwise unresponsive, may grimace at the stick of a needle. But in others, even that indication may be absent. This the doctors and nurses themselves will often acknowledge. One Outerboro nurse, for example, had just told me that the treatment of one patient "was a farce. The poor man, we were torturing him." Yet, when I asked her if she knew he was in pain, she answered simply, "I can't say. I don't know." A resident was even less sure:

I don't know what it's like to have a tube in your throat. I think to some extent you'll acclimate to it. . . . If they're alert, they're always sedated. I think nine out of ten people with a tube have to have some form of sedation. . . . If someone's brain-dead and has no withdrawal, clearly drawing a blood isn't going to make any difference.

Torture is a strong word. It suggests deep feelings. Yet the ICU doctors and ICU nurses are not sure how much pain they are inflicting or even, in some instances, whether they are inflicting any pain at all. What they are sure of is that their own efforts are futile. "The whole point of those of us who

3. See Elaine Scarry, *The Body in Pain* (New York: Oxford University Press, 1985). For a general discussion of physicians' and nurses' orientation to pain in acute care hospitals, see Shizuko Y. Fagerhaugh and Anselm Strauss, *The Politics of Pain Management* (Menlo Park, CA: Addison-Wesley, 1977).

don't want to be aggressive," one resident explained, "is that it doesn't make any difference in the end." And what seems likely is that the depth of feelings emerges from this sense of futility rather than from the infliction of pain on patients. This is not to question the sincerity of the doctors' and nurses' comments or the degree to which they are genuinely concerned with the consequences of their actions. It is to suggest that, whatever else, torture is, in part, a self-reflective concept.

Treating incurable patients is not only painful to the patient but painful to the ICU staff itself. Consider a nurse's comments about an incurable patient who had been in the Outerboro unit for many weeks and had then been resuscitated. "I just don't understand it," she told me. "To me it's just so wrong. It's just so torturous. So when I feel strong, when I'm not drained, when I'm not here four days in a row, I can go in and I can provide support and provide care and not feel so drained. But day after day it really gets to me." From discussing a procedure that was "torturous" to a patient, she moved quickly to discussing the effects of that procedure on herself: "Day after day it really gets to me." A resident made the same point even more explicitly: "The physical act of doing all sorts of lines and things, I think that is what cheechee refers to. We are torturing ourselves by doing that." Torture refers not just to the suffering of patients but also to the suffering of doctors and nurses.

The treatment of incurable patients is torture to the ICU staff not because it involves more work. Incurable patients usually require less work than do those with a chance of recovery. Such treatment is torture because it marks the limits of medicine.[4] The treatment of incurable patients marks the limits of medicine, in part, in that it is a reminder to doctors and nurses that the ability to cure is sometimes beyond the technical skills of their vocation. Even more important, though, it marks the limits of doctors and nurses to set their own agenda. *"You have no choice but to torture them,"* one resident told me, "because that's what they're there for, to be intensely monitored, which means drawing bloods from them and sticking [them with] those huge needles."

More specifically, it is my impression that the term "torture" is invoked more often by those with the least control over treatment decisions. The term is used far less frequently at Countryside than at Outerboro, where the prohibition on withdrawing respirator care often leaves physicians and nurses

4. For a superb discussion of the use of the term "Gomer" following similar lines of analysis, see Deborah B. Liederman and Jean-Anne Grisso, "The Gomer Phenomenon," *Journal of Health and Social Behavior* 26 (1985): 222–32.

convinced that critical decisions have been taken out of their hands alto-gether. Moreover, although I do not have strong evidence, the term appears to be used at both hospitals more frequently and more broadly by those at the bottom of the medical hierarchy. Unlike physicians, nurses will occasion-ally extend the term to include the treatment of patients with some chance of recovery, a use absent among physicians. Interns use the term more fre-quently than do residents; and residents, more frequently than attendings.

Although the doctors and nurses did not themselves make the observa-tion, they in fact invoked the concept of torture only in those cases in which they felt that an obligation to treat had been imposed on them. In not a single instance was the notion of "torture" used by a doctor or nurse in a circum-stance in which he or she could claim effective participation in the decision to treat. For the entire staff—attendings, housestaff, and nurses alike—the obligation to treat may be imposed at the insistence of a private physician, by the wishes of the patient's family, or by a perceived legal responsibility. But nurses and housestaff also face obligations that the attendings do not. For nurses, the obligation to treat is imposed by the medical staff. A nurse:

A nurse knows the torture the patient is going through and can give at least the pa-tient's reaction of it in terms of resistance, in terms of depression, in terms of all these things which I think are overlooked. I think a nurse has to be brought in on it—how the nurse feels about it, but more so from the patient's point of view. But I think that doctors rarely ask nurses how they feel about caring for these people who are ob-viously dying and the physician writes an order, especially on these isolation patients.

For the housestaff, the obligation to treat may be imposed by attendings.

Mr. Andrews, a 30-year-old man with probable AIDS, had been transferred to the unit late at night in respiratory distress. Despite his difficulty breathing, he had re-fused intubation, a choice that both the attending and resident on duty were prepared to respect. But the next morning, the attendings insisted on intubation, regardless of Mr. Andrews's wishes. While they were examining the patient in his room, the resi-dent who had been in charge of the case took me aside: "Something happens to attendings when they become attendings." Some months later, in an interview, the resident remembered the case vividly: "He was clearly just a frightened man. And what he'd been through was like torture, and for no end, really."

If nurses use the term "torture" more frequently than housestaff and house-staff more frequently than attendings, it is because "torture" is an expression of powerlessness.

Torture, then, marks the social, as well as the more narrowly technical, limits of medical practice. It expresses not simply the limits of medical tech-nology but also the limits of doctors and nurses, individually and collectively, to determine when treatment should be withheld. The treatment of incurable patients becomes "torture" because it challenges assumptions fundamental to the occupational identity of doctors and nurses. For the doctor, it makes clear the tension between compassion and the compulsive effort that is in other circumstances admirable. But, more important, for both doctors and nurses, it shakes an already fragile sense of control. Incurable illness is a reproach to medicine, a reminder to doctors and nurses that, in the end, they cannot control death. The obligation to treat incurable patients is even worse: It is a reminder to doctors and nurses that they cannot control even their own efforts.

9

Uncertainty, the Social Organization of Medicine, and Limitation of Treatment

The point bears repeating. At Outerboro, physicians limit at least some form of potentially life-prolonging treatment for roughly one in every seven patients discharged from the Intensive Care Unit; at Countryside, they limit for one in four. Yet it is the general consensus of physicians in both units—albeit with occasional exceptions—that they do too much. An Outerboro resident:

I think there is a small number of people, but a very small number, who benefit in the unit. . . . I think we do a little bit of good. But I think we do a lot of bad. I think we do a lot of bad because there are people who are artificially prolonged way beyond . . . any reasonable prognosis.

A Countryside resident made a similar observation: "I think we err far too much on the side of doing too much rather than too little. I can't think of one instance where I felt we hadn't done enough." Physicians, in their own view, overtreat. Why?

Both the law and the general consensus of medical ethics insist that treatment may be withheld or withdrawn only from patients who are on a clearly "terminal" course. Anything else would verge on homicide or, at the very least, active assistance in suicide, a practice which is both legally proscribed and, according to most thought on the subject, ethically unacceptable. Before limiting treatment, physicians want to be certain they understand the course of the patient's disease, that he or she is, in fact, incurable, irrevocably beyond the help of medical intervention. But certainty, a difficult enough state of mind to achieve in any circumstances, is particularly elusive in medicine.

Whatever the pretensions of medicine in this respect (and they are, for the most part, fairly modest), medicine is not a theoretical science. Unlike chemistry or physics, medicine does not set as its task the formulation of general, abstract laws. Rather, medicine is an applied science, one that takes general principles and brings them to bear on particular cases. But the particular cases are always messier and more complex than the general principles, filled with qualifications, ambiguities, and uncertainties.

Faced with these uncertainties, the physicians at Outerboro and Country-side will often retreat to a language of probability, suggesting, for example, that they are "95 percent" or "98 percent" or "99 percent" sure that a patient is irretrievably incurable. But a language of probability is fundamentally incompatible with any notion of certainty. Moreover, even the probabilities, as many physicians themselves readily acknowledge in more reflective moments, are at best very rough estimates. As one Outerboro attending, Mark, explained:

No one has the numbers. You can't be a scientist and say 90 percent. One or two diseases here people have worked out numbers and things like how much lung can be removed from somebody before they can't breathe on their own. But other than that example I can't think of anything else. . . . No one has that kind of data. For the similar patient, there are so many variables that to have enough numbers with each of the variables [is] absurd.

Despite—or, perhaps, because of—their pervasive uncertainty, the Outerboro and Countryside physicians hold themselves to strict standards before limiting treatment. As Mark continued, "If I'm pretty sure, it means I'm 90 percent sure, which means one out of ten times I could be wrong. . . . If you're dealing with somebody and one out of ten times you're wrong and they really could have a long life afterwards, that's a gamble I'm certainly not going to make." In a similar spirit, one Outerboro intern described the uncertainties he felt in withholding treatment from a patient with metastatic cancer:

What if he had woken up, really woken up, and we had been saying, "Oh, he has no prognosis. His mental status is out. . . . Forget it"? What if we had been doing that and he had woken up? That would have been horrible. . . . I don't have enough sense and experience with these things to really gauge them. All I can say is . . . "Mr. Finn [another patient] is unresponsive. He has all these millions of medical problems. It doesn't look like he's going to get better . . . and he's just going to die." I was perfectly right in his case, and I was right in Mendoza's case [yet another patient]. But I could have been 100 percent wrong. . . . What if he had woken up and said, "Hey, let's go home. Let me go to my daughter's wedding in a month"?

What the physicians are looking for is certainty about a prognosis. But prognostic certainty depends, in turn, on diagnostic certainty. Consider, for example, the following cases:

Mr. Ouimette had been in the Outerboro unit for over a week and was deteriorating quickly. From the time of his admission the ICU staff had been "almost certain" he was suffering from AIDS, a preliminary diagnosis suggested by his homosexual history and confirmed by a wide range of clinical symptoms. Nonetheless, the ICU staff were unable to confirm their diagnosis definitively with laboratory tests. When one of the residents raised the possibility of withholding cardiopulmonary resuscitation, she did so tentatively: "We don't really know where he stands, so it's hard to discuss it with the family." An attending concurred: "We can't [withhold CPR] if we don't have a neuro diagnosis, and we don't know if he can come back. . . . I think we will agree he's likely to have AIDS, but I don't think we can [withhold CPR] unless we know he has something irreversible."

Mr. Pike had been admitted to the Countryside ICU after a cardiopulmonary arrest at home. He was unresponsive, and a CAT scan showed that 80 to 90 percent of one lung was filled with a tumor. John, who was the attending on the day of Pike's admission, pressed to make him DNR and raised the possibility of a terminal wean. But the next afternoon, when Ken returned to the unit, he disagreed: "How could you make him a DNR without knowing why he coded? . . . What right do you have to make him DNR just because he has a tumor . . . ? If I came as a witness in a court of law, I would destroy this case for the simple reason you haven't made a definitive diagnosis of hypoxic encephalopathy. . . . You can't make a DNR until five days after [the diagnosis].

Despite it all, certainty is not a chimera, at least as a state of mind. (Whether certainty is ever objectively possible is an altogether different matter, about which skepticism is well warranted.) Confronted with enough evidence, equipped with a confirmed diagnosis, understanding the underlying logic of a disease process, having seen sufficient patients in sufficiently similar circumstances, both the Outerboro and the Countryside physicians are prepared to declare themselves certain a patient cannot survive. But, as should be apparent by this point, certainty is not easily achieved, even as a state of mind.

Uncertainty is pervasive, and, combined with physicians' unwillingness to withdraw treatments once begun, its consequences are far-reaching. So as not to miss a case in which their failure to treat might cost the life of a patient, ICU physicians err more often on the side of treating patients whose lives they cannot save.[1] Because they are uncertain of what will eventually happen, physicians admit patients to the ICU, place them on respirators, begin them

1. On the difference between what are called "Type I" and "Type II" errors in medicine, see Thomas Scheff, "Decision Rules, Types of Error, and Their Consequences in Medical Diagnosis," *Behavioral Science* 8 (1963): 97–107; Diana Crane, *The Sanctity of Social Life* (New York: Russell Sage, 1975), pp. 203–6; and Jeanne Harley Guilleman and Lynda Lytle Holmstrom, *Mixed Blessings: Intensive Care for Newborns* (New York: Oxford University Press, 1986), pp. 125–30.

on pressors. Later, when they are more certain that there is no hope of recovery, physicians (especially at Outerboro) are unwilling to send the patient out, turn off the respirator, discontinue pressors. Uncertainty leads the physicians down a road with no exit.

Uncertainty, as Renee Fox has observed, emerges, in part, from "limitations in current medical knowledge. There are innumerable questions to which no physician, however well trained, can as yet provide answers." [2] Such limitations, by themselves, would make the work of ICU physicians difficult enough. But to them are added uncertainties which emerge, much more directly, from the social organization of medicine.

First, uncertainties emerge from an emphasis in the organization of contemporary hospitals on familiarity with techniques rather than familiarity with patients. In the hospitals that provide critical care, particularly if they are urban and even more if they are teaching hospitals, doctors are often called on to make life and death decisions for patients they are seeing for the first time. In the ICU and in the Emergency Room, where many of the decisions are made that result in intubation and transfer to the unit, doctors must often treat patients before they have had the chance to collect a history or review records. According to an Outerboro resident: "You've got to understand that someone rolls into the Emergency Room . . . you've never met before in your entire life . . . and you've got thirty seconds to decide whether you're going to intubate them or not. And that's probably half the cases." Even after a patient has been in the unit, the constant rotation of housestaff and attendings may create uncertainty. An Outerboro resident again:

People rotate every two weeks in the unit. So I think every two weeks you get a new group of bright-eyed, bushy-tailed people that come in. . . . They really don't get to know the patient and the . . . chronicity of the patient's disease for at least several days. So if someone should arrest who should really be let go on the first day, I think there's a high percentage of his being resuscitated. You just don't know the patient that well.

Prognostic and diagnostic certainty require not only a knowledge of a patient's current condition but also an ability to compare that condition with a baseline, with the patient's usual condition. The social organization of the urban teaching hospital, which throws doctor and patient together as virtual strangers, denies doctors that ability.

Second, even when physicians have some knowledge of a patient's prior medical condition, they are often unaware of that patient's wishes as they

2. Renee Fox, "Training for Uncertainty," in Robert Merton, George Reader, and Patricia Kendall, eds., *The Student Physician*, p. 208 (Cambridge, MA: Harvard University Press, 1957).

bear on aggressive treatment. Although the wishes of the patient or the patient's surrogate are at best an ambiguous influence on doctors' willingness to limit treatment (about which, much more later), they are a consideration nonetheless. But many physicians are uncomfortable discussing such issues, particularly when a patient appears to be doing well. As a result, if the patient does deteriorate, the medical staff are often left unprepared. To the residents who are left to care for dying patients, this is a source of considerable anger. A Countryside intern: "They call up and there's this guy on the floor and he's in respiratory failure with pneumonia, COPD [chronic obstructive pulmonary disease]. Nobody has made the decision not to intubate this guy when it [an arrest] happens, so he gets in." An Outerboro resident:

It's ridiculous. The most frequent is . . . the oncology patients. . . . They just don't address it. Two of the oncologists, several of the oncologists here are like that. . . . This guy is on a general medical floor, for some reason becomes septic or whatever, has nothing, no chance of reversal, and gets intubated because the question had not been addressed. . . . It happens frequently with private patients here where it's the fault of the private physician, the private attending. It happened earlier in the year more frequently with house officers.

To the uncertainties of diagnosis and prognosis are added the uncertainties of the patient's wishes. This is a matter not of the limitations of medical science but of the limitations of medical practice.

Third, and most important, uncertainty is exacerbated by a long-standing system of decision making that emphasizes the responsibility of individual physicians. Certainty as an individual state of mind does not require unanimity. But certainty as a social fact does. Thus, the insistent dissent of a single physician from what is otherwise a consensus is sufficient to establish doubt. To be sure, individual physicians may hold, even against a dissenting voice, to their own conviction that a patient is irretrievably dying. Doctors can cling to their own beliefs as stubbornly as anyone else. But from the point of view of the group, considering certainty as a social phenomenon (rather than simply a phenomenon of individual belief), the dissent of a single physician is sufficient to introduce uncertainty. As one Outerboro resident explained:

There are nine people on the housestaff and attending team. And, really, you have to satisfy, in a sense, all nine people, all of whom have different ideas and different thresholds for declaring a case hopeless. So, in a sense, you have to go up to a fairly high level on the hopeless scale. . . . Anybody can say yes to keep going. It's sort of like the U.N. It has to be unanimous.

It should come as no surprise that a private physician or a consultant can insist successfully on treatment even when the entire ICU staff believes that treatment is pointless.

Mr. Carey, who had first come into the hospital for elective surgery, had been admitted to the Countryside ICU after a cardiac arrest. After the first day of Carey's unit admission, Ken was prepared to pull back: "The first twenty-four hours of admission you have to be a full court press. Now this guy has nonrefractory septic shock. . . . His prognosis is not good." As the intern explained that Mr. Carey was continuing to receive large doses of dopamine and levophed, two powerful vasopressors, the resident wondered out loud, "Why are we doing these things?" The next day the situation was even worse, and Ken described the situation as hopeless. But Carey's intern reported, "We're still a full court press on him." When Ken objected, the intern explained, "It's what came down from the attendings." And the resident added, "This is where Strait [Carey's neurologist] is extremely poor. He tells us zero chance and writes extremely poor in the chart." Ken: "Don't talk to me about it." Mr. Carey died later that day, but despite his continued treatment and with neither any treatment withdrawn nor a Do Not Resuscitate order written.

Slightly more surprising is the ability of a resident to insist on treatment against the objections of the remainder of the ICU team.

Mr. Tidrow, a 38-year-old homeless alcoholic, was unresponsive and had not stopped bleeding after numerous transfusions. One of the attendings was prepared to place a limit on the Outerboro ICU's efforts: "I think we should decide how much blood we should give him." One of the residents was even blunter: "We should stop." But Sarah, one of the other residents, disagreed: "I think he's already slowed down. He's a young guy. Support him fully." Both attendings argued with Sarah as did the other two residents. But Sarah was adamant: "Support means transfusions. It's as important to this guy as his respirator." The team agreed to additional transfusions.

Even more surprising is the ability of a physician with no official responsibility for a patient to insist on treatment, as in the following case, also drawn from Outerboro.

Mr. Figueroa, a 57-year-old man with alcoholic cirrhosis, had become unresponsive. After a discussion with Mr. Figueroa's family, his private physician had recommended that he receive no further platelets (a type of blood transfusion), no dialysis, no vasopressors, and no cardiopulmonary resuscitation in the event of an arrest. The ICU staff agreed. But a consultant on the case disagreed: "Apparently he was very close to death eight or nine years ago and came back. This man is made of very good protoplasm." The attendings continued to believe that Mr. Figueroa could not be helped: "We don't have anything to offer him." Nonetheless they agreed to additional transfusions, as did Mr. Figueroa's private physician, although he, too, "personally felt differently." (Despite these efforts, Mr. Figueroa died two days later.)

Medicine, as virtually all who observe it have argued, relies on the good judgment and good faith of individual physicians.[3] In solo practice and even in many group practices, where few other controls are available, individual responsibility, however imperfect, is the only safeguard of sound medical practice. But the individual responsibility that is a necessity in those circumstances takes on a very different meaning in the ICU. To limit treatment, the ICU physicians require certainty. But certainty requires consensus and an emphasis on the responsibility of individual physicians makes that consensus all the harder to achieve. Compared to most settings in which medicine is practiced, intensive care units emphasize collective decisions. Yet, even in the ICU, medicine lacks the means for imposing a collective will on dissenting physicians. The individual responsibility that is, in other settings, the basis for making decisions becomes, in the ICU, the means through which decisions are blocked.

3. Although they disagree as to the sources and consequences of this reliance, see, for example, Charles Bosk, *Forgive and Remember: Managing Medical Failure* (Chicago: University of Chicago Press, 1979), and Eliot Freidson, *Doctoring Together: A Study of Professional Social Control* (Chicago: University of Chicago Press, 1975).

10

Withholding, Withdrawing, and
the "Terminal" Patient

Uncertainty limits the discretion of physicians. But it does not eliminate it. In the face of uncertainty, physicians struggle to maintain discretion. They do so, in part, by conceptualizing both the course of illness and the types of treatment in terms that allow for wide latitude in judgments as to what constitutes "appropriate" action. This strategy is evident in the ways physicians conceptualize "terminal" illness. It is also evident in the distinction they make between "aggressive" and "unaggressive" treatments.

The Terminal Patient

In his *Passing On*, David Sudnow levels perhaps as damaging a charge against medicine as one can imagine. Physicians, according to Sudnow, are less likely to attempt resuscitating

the suicide victim, the dope addict, the known prostitute, the assailant in a crime of violence, the vagrant, the known wife-beater, and, generally, those persons whose moral characters are considered reproachable. . . . If one anticipates having a critical heart attack, he had best keep himself well-dressed and his breath clean.[1]

Physicians, contends Sudnow, allow their own values, particularly as they shape views of their patients' character, to intrude on nothing less than their decisions whether or not to treat critically ill patients. This is very much not the role envisioned for doctors in either the law or medical ethics.

As I pointed out in the previous chapter, both the law and most discussions in medical ethics insist that treatment may be withheld or withdrawn only from already incurable patients. In this sense, the decision to limit treat-

---

1. David Sudnow, *Passing On: The Social Organization of Dying* (Englewood Cliffs, NJ: Prentice Hall, 1967), p. 105.

ment—at least on the doctor's part—would seem to depend on a fairly straightforward question: Is the patient, despite the best efforts of medicine, on a course that will lead inevitably to death? This question is, of course, sometimes technically complex. But it is, at least apparently, morally simple.

In this chapter, I argue that neither Sudnow's biting criticism of physicians nor the high hopes expressed in the law and medical ethics provide an adequate description of medical practice in intensive care. On the one hand, I found little evidence to support Sudnow's claim that doctors limit treatment on the basis of their own judgments about the "social worth" of their patients.[2] On the other hand, I found considerable evidence that doctors' judgments, though based on considerations other than those identified by Sudnow, do intrude on their decision-making process. These judgments are not about the moral character of patients but about the task of medicine. They are judgments about what it is worthwhile for physicians to do, regardless of the character of the patient. In particular, I found that physicians at Countryside limit treatment more frequently than do those at Outerboro. This difference represents a difference in the moral stance of the two units. It is an expression of their collective values. But it is not expressed as such. To the contrary, doctors at both Countryside and Outerboro articulate strikingly similar principles in their decisions to limit treatment. At both hospitals these principles appear to rest on exclusively technical judgments. And at both hospitals physicians insist that they limit treatment only for terminally ill patients. But they in fact ascribe very different meanings to the concept of "terminal." Thus, while assuming a position of strict technical expertise and value neutrality, physicians, in effect, apply their moral judgments to matters of nothing less than the maintenance of life itself.

In the units at both hospitals, physicians advocate limiting treatment of patients whose conditions are ultimately incurable—and *only* from patients whose conditions are incurable. Consider, first, a Countryside case:

Mr. Charles, a 62-year-old nursing home resident, had been admitted to the Countryside ICU with severe emphysema, an exacerbation of his Chronic Obstructive Pulmonary Disease, and bronchospasms. Mr. Charles had been intubated as soon as he arrived in the unit, and several attempts to extubate him had failed. After a week of failed attempts, one of the interns reported during rounds that Mr. Charles's disease was now "end stage," that he was about to be made DNR, and that there was a possi-

2. For other research critical of Sudnow along the same lines, see Diana Crane, *The Sanctity of Social Life* (New York: Russell Sage, 1975). I should, however, acknowledge the possibility that Sudnow's research presents an accurate portrayal of emergency rooms even if it does not pertain to intensive care units.

bility of either a terminal wean or a transfer to the floor with a fixed ventilator setting. John, the attending, wanted to be sure: "And we agree with this assessment, that he's end of road?" The resident answered that she, in any event, did agree. John persisted: "Is there any reversible process?" The intern answered that there was not. John still persisted: "We glibly use the term end stage. Is he really end stage?" The intern insisted that he was. Mr. Charles's private physician wrote a DNR order that afternoon with the full agreement of the ICU staff.

Consider, also, a case at Outerboro:

Mr. Salvucci was transferred directly to the Outerboro ICU from the Emergency Room after a presumed drug overdose. He was unresponsive and an emergency CT scan (in effect, an X-ray of the brain) showed cerebral edema. One of the attendings summed up the situation: "The practical reality is that we're faced with a man whose chances for recovery are practically nil. Has any of this been broached with the wife?" When one of the residents answered that he had, in fact, discussed withholding therapies with Mrs. Salvucci, the second attending objected strenuously: "Am I missing something? Do we know the diagnosis? Before we write this guy off as dead, don't we want to know what happened?" Although the first attending continued to think that Mr. Salvucci wasn't "going to make it," he was nonetheless convinced: "He warrants support, [at least] until we've confirmed our initial impression."

In both cases the principle is the same. Limit treatment only if the course of the disease is clearly incurable. There seems, in neither formulation, any place for physicians' values.

Because physicians advocate limiting treatment for incurable patients, certain diseases whose courses result in almost certain death provoke especially frequent discussions of at least the possibility of limiting treatment. Foremost among these diseases are AIDS and some types of cancer. Although physicians discussed limiting treatment in one-quarter of all the Outerboro ICU cases, they discussed it in eight of ten AIDS cases. (They eventually limited treatment in four of these cases.) Similarly, they discussed limiting treatment in eighteen of thirty cancer cases (and actually limited treatment in eleven). Although physicians discussed limiting treatment in one-third of all Countryside cases, they raised the issue in three of six AIDS cases (and actually limited treatment in two) and in five of nine cancer cases (and actually limited treatment in four). The frequency with which physicians at both Outerboro and Countryside suggest limiting treatment of AIDS and cancer patients poses, however, no special moral problems. Physicians do not advocate limiting treatment of patients with these diseases because of any special horror for cancer patients or any special distaste for AIDS patients. Rather, physicians at both Outerboro and Countryside are more likely to suggest limiting treatment of AIDS and cancer patients than

of other patients as a simple application of what remains a technical judgment. Whatever the complexities of other diseases, virtually all AIDS patients and many types of cancer patients face a certain death.[3]

Whether a patient is considered terminal is not, however, simply a judgment about the disease itself. It is also a judgment about what might be called
the patient's career in that disease. Thus, the physicians at both Outerboro
and Countryside are more sympathetic to withholding treatment from an
AIDS patient hospitalized for the second time with pneumocystis carinii
pneumonia (PCP, a pneumonia characteristic of AIDS) than one hospitalized for the first time.

Mr. Espinoza, a 32-year-old intravenous drug user, was admitted to the Countryside
ICU with pneumocystis carinii pneumonia. After hearing the case presentation, Ken's
(the attending's) first question was, "Is this the first time he's been in the ICU?" The
intern answered that it was the first time he had been in the hospital. Ken: "Okay.
That's different; his prognosis is good."

An Outerboro resident articulated the same principle:

I think basically it's been shown that, in patients with their first bout of PCP, there's a
fairly good chance that they can be gotten over it and survive. And since these are
young people, you may be able to give them a year or two more of life. I think in the
first bout they deserve the unit bed. It's very hard to make hard and fast rules because
these are young people. After the first bout, I'm not sure that they should go to the
unit.

Similarly, physicians at both Outerboro and Countryside are more likely to
consider withholding future treatments from a patient after a trial of dialysis,
if it becomes clear that dialysis will not resolve an underlying problem, than
before that trial. And a patient who has not wakened from a coma after a

---

3. For a different view of the high incidence of DNR orders among AIDS and cancer patients, see Robert M. Wachter, John M. Luce, Norman Hearst, and Bernard Lo, "Decisions
about Resuscitation: Inequities among Patients with Different Diseases but Similar Prognoses,"
Annals of Internal Medicine 111 (1989): 525–32. Wachter and his colleagues show, convincingly,
that at three San Francisco teaching hospitals AIDS and lung cancer patients are made DNR
more often than patients with severe congestive heart failure or cirrhosis of the liver accompanied by a history of esophageal varices, both groups with prognoses as bleak as those of patients
with AIDS and cancer. However, as Wachter and his colleagues acknowledge, some of the difference may be accounted for by physicians' belief that more effective therapies are available for
heart failure and cirrhosis than are available for either AIDS or lung cancer. Some of the difference may also be accounted for (especially in San Francisco) by the varying expectations of
patients in the different diagnostic groups rather than by the intentions of physicians. And, finally, the Wachter study was designed to identify differences in treatment among patients with
similar prognoses. It does not (and was not meant to) dispute my claim that the primary explanation of different treatment decisions is variation in prognosis.

week is treated very differently from one who has been in a coma for only a day.

Age, Social Worth, and Quality of Life

Distinctions among diseases or among patients' courses in those diseases are, of course, primarily technical. But there are three other types of distinctions that physicians might make and each much more clearly involves value-laden judgments: distinctions between older and younger patients, distinctions on the basis of the patient's character, and distinctions on the basis of quality of life. Age is perhaps the most complex of these distinctions. On the one hand, advocating the limitation of treatment for older patients represents, in part, a technical judgment. Age, even apart from other indicators, may imply a lower likelihood of surviving the rigors of ICU treatment. On the other hand, advocating the limitation of treatment for older patients may also represent a judgment about the value of life to an 80-year-old or 90-year-old. Certainly, physicians at both Outerboro and Countryside will occasionally express their reservations about treating older patients aggressively.

Mr. Marrero, a 93-year-old, had been transferred to the Countryside ICU from a nearby hospital after his gastrointestinal bleed had been complicated by severe kidney failure. Discussing him on rounds, Ken suggested, "I wouldn't do that much. . . . The fact that he has mental status change, the fact that he has renal failure, the fact that he has hypertension, his mortality is 60 percent." A resident disagreed: "That's not so bad." But an intern pointed out: "You add in that he's 93, and you don't treat." And Ken assented, "That's right."

The difficult question, however, is whether physicians limit the treatment of older patients more frequently than of younger ones, *apart* from age-related judgments about the probability of survival. In fact, physicians sentiments notwithstanding, there is little evidence that they do. To be sure, if we look at all the patients discharged from the units at Outerboro and Countryside, the patients whose treatment was limited are significantly older than those whose treatment was not (62.4 to 57.7 at Outerboro, 64.4 to 54.8 at Countryside). But much of this difference can be accounted for by differences in the mortality rates of older and younger patients. As a result, if we limit our comparison to patients who died without leaving the hospital, the differences are significantly reduced. Of eighty-seven patients at Outerboro who died without leaving the hospital—a means of controlling for mortality—the average age of those whose treatment was limited was 61.8 compared to 59.3

for those whose treatment was not limited. Of the forty patients who died at Countryside, the average age of those whose treatment was limited was 64.1 compared to 62.9 for those whose treatment was not limited. All this hardly constitutes definitive evidence that physicians do not consider age, apart from prognosis, in decisions to limit treatment. But it does *suggest* that they do not. And it is altogether possible that, with more sophisticated measures of survival probabilities, the difference would disappear altogether.

Decision making on the basis of considerations about the character of patients would involve a clear intrusion of values. Judgments about patients' character—or about "social worth" and an assumed contribution to society—are made routinely. Moreover, whether a physician likes a patient— more likely in the case of a "solid citizen," less likely in the case of a drug user or heavy drinker—may subtly influence the efforts he or she brings to bear in a case. "I think there is a bias," an Outerboro resident acknowledged, "against people who are sociopathic and engage in self-destructive behavior." "We don't like noncompliant people," another resident told me. "They don't do what we tell them, and we know that." At times, a patient's habits may contribute to the difficulty of treating effectively. In the case of alcoholics and drug users, in particular, the very habits that make physicians question their character also make it unlikely that the meliorative efforts available to the ICU staff will have much long-term success. And in these circumstances the objections to active treatment become more explicit. "Do people," an Outerboro attending asked rhetorically, "whose illness is a result of their abusing themselves deserve the same level of care as people who don't do that? Obviously a person who is a civil libertarian would say that everybody should get the same. But I'm not sure that I agree with that." But even these objections, however deeply felt by individual physicians, are rarely acted on. When considerations of character or social worth are raised on rounds—as they are from time to time—they are just as quickly dismissed as the basis for decisions whether or not to limit treatment.

Mr. Fisher had been admitted to the Outerboro unit with a drug overdose after his girlfriend had found him lying, unresponsive, in their apartment with a needle in his arm. When a neurologist, Dan Samson, came by to assess Fisher, he asked: "What was he before?" Dennis, the attending, answered, "We didn't know him. . . . He was a drug user. . . . He's somebody's son, somebody's husband. He was a person." Samson persisted, "Was he a criminal?" But Dennis persisted, too: "Would it be different?" After Samson had left, Dennis told the staff, "He just likes to stir things up." Fisher was treated with all available means until his wife requested that he be made DNR.

Even in cases like that of Mr. Fisher, in which patients clearly, explicitly, and immediately brought illness on themselves, ICU doctors do not convert their judgments about the patient's style of life into a decision to limit treatment. As Mark, an Outerboro attending, put it, "I can't think of ever seeing someone say, 'This guy's the scum of the earth. Let's not save him.' I've seen a lot of guys who were shot by the cops while they shot someone else, and they have gotten the same care as if they had been the policemen themselves." Judgments about character may subtly influence decisions whether or not to limit treatment. But such judgments exercise, at most, a marginal influence.

Even more tempting to physicians than judgments about character are judgments about quality of life. While judgments about character involve more or less explicit moralizing, considerations about quality of life seem compassionate and patient centered. Here, too, physicians are anything but bashful in expressing their views that quality of life should be considered in deciding whether to limit treatment. One Countryside intern, for example, told me that he considered quality of life "all the time."

What was the person like outside, before they come into the ICU? Are they functional people? Are they sitting in a nursing home somewhere? Are they unresponsive and incontinent? I have strong beliefs about quality of life.

Such considerations open the way to a wide range of explicit value judgments. They open the way, for example, to judgments about whether the life of a profoundly retarded man is worth living, about whether a physically incapacitated widow's life is worth living, whether life is worth living without the ability to travel or eat certain kinds of food or do virtually anything else. But whatever their own views about which lives are worth living and which not, the physicians at both Outerboro and Countryside are remarkably slow to impose such views on patients. Rather, physicians at both hospitals typically limit their judgments about quality of life to a very circumscribed distinction.

One Outerboro attending, for example, was prepared to propose the possibility of regaining a "reasonable life-style" as a standard for aggressive treatment. But when I pressed him to explain what he meant by a "reasonable life-style," he said: "From my point of view, I think [it is having] a certain clarity, mental clarity, that would allow you to communicate with your family and friends." A resident was even more explicit in explaining his standard of a "salvageable" patient:

What I would call a minimal functional capacity, meaning that they're able to interact in a meaningful way with other human beings. I don't care if they can't feed themselves or are bed-bound. . . . I think . . . the best definition would be someone who can just have a meaningful interaction with somebody else.

In a sense, these comments are not a judgment about quality of life at all. Rather, they represent an extension of the meaning of death—albeit a somewhat metaphorical one—from simple physiological death to a death of consciousness.[45] As another Outerboro attending explained, on virtually the first day of my research, "I always ask about the head first, because if the head isn't there, the rest doesn't matter." His sentiment was repeated routinely at both hospitals.

Mr. Carmine had been transferred to the Countryside ICU from a nearby hospital with an upper gastrointestinal bleed, complicated by hypertension and renal failure. The housestaff treated Carmine's renal failure aggressively, but their attending was critical: "You're saving this man's kidney while he's dying. . . . You were ignoring the overall physiology in an effort to get one system working. . . . We'd rather lose his kidney than his head."

The notion that death consists not only of physiological death but also of a death of consciousness does, to be sure, involve physicians in a type of value judgment—in a judgment that certain kinds of life are worth living and that others are not. Thus, the Outerboro and Countryside physicians introduce an element of values into their conception of the terminal patient, extending it from physiological death to death of consciousness. But at the same time, they quickly pull back from this lapse in their stance of disinterested technical expertise. They do not generalize their distinction between patients with consciousness and patients without to other dimensions of quality of life. For the most part, their question remains an explicitly technical one (albeit one framed, implicitly, by fundamental values). Given that only

4. The permanent loss of consciousness should not be confused with "brain death." Brain death is not a type of death but a criterion of death. It refers to the loss of all brain functions, including brain stem and cranial reflexes. By permanent loss of consciousness I mean only the loss or severe impairment of cognitive abilities, which is compatible with some spontaneous cardiac and respiratory functions.

5. My findings parallel those reported by Crane in her study *Sanctity of Social Life*, which is based on physicians' survey responses to vignettes. According to Crane, the operational meaning of a death of consciousness is typically the patient's inability to engage in some kind of human interaction: "Physicians respond to the chronically ill or terminally ill patient not simply in terms of physiological definitions of illness but also in terms of the extent to which the patient is capable of interacting with others. The treatable patient is one who can interact or who has the potential to act in a meaningful way with others in his environment. The physically damaged salvageable patient whose life can be maintained for a considerable period of time is more likely to be treated actively than the severely brain-damaged patient" (p. 199).

life with consciousness is worth living—and disregarding any other criteria of quality of life—can "meaningful" life be restored?

The Meaning of "Terminal"

Because physicians limit treatment only of patients who are already dying, those patients rarely survive their hospital stay. At Outerboro, of the thirty-six patients whose treatment physicians limited, 61 percent died without leaving the unit and an additional 31 percent died without leaving the hospital. In contrast, over three-quarters of those patients whose treatment physicians did not discuss limiting survived their hospital stay. At Countryside, of the thirty-two patients whose treatment physicians limited, half died in the unit and another 28 percent without leaving the hospital. In contrast, over 90 percent of those patients whose treatment physicians did not discuss limiting survived their hospital stay.

Because physicians limit treatment only of patients who are already dying, limiting treatment confirms—and perhaps speeds—death. But it does not cause death. Despite the very large differences in survival rates between those patients whose treatment was limited and those for whom it was not even considered, we should not imagine that this difference can be accounted for by the decision to limit treatment. If it were, we would also expect a large difference in death rates between those from whom treatment was in fact limited and those for whom it was discussed but not limited. But the difference in the death rate of those patients from whom treatment was in fact limited is only slightly higher than the death rate among those patients for whom limiting treatment was discussed but decided against (92 percent compared to 86 percent at Outerboro, 78 percent compared to 71 percent at Countryside), statistically insignificant differences.[6]

Still, when all is said and done, there remains a striking difference between Countryside and Outerboro. While the Countryside physicians limit treatment for nearly one-third of all unit patients, the Outerboro physicians limit treatment for less than one in six—even though their patient population

---

6. These findings are confirmed by Charlson's considerably more sophisticated study of mortality and morbidity rates at New York Hospital-Cornell Medical Center: "Within prognostically similar groups . . . patients in the not-full intervention group did not have significantly higher mortality rates than those for whom full intervention was preferred." Mary E. Charlson, Frederic L. Sax, Ronald MacKenzie, Suzanne D. Fields, Robert L. Braham, and R. Gordon Douglas, Jr., "Resuscitation: How Do We Decide?" *Journal of the American Medical Association* 255 (1986): 1320.

is equally or more critically ill. This difference cannot be accounted for by any insistence on different principles at the two hospitals. At both, physicians insist that they limit treatment only for terminal patients. Rather, it is a difference in the application of a principle. Most important, the Countryside physicians limit treatment on the basis of a looser standard of terminal illness than the standard at Outerboro. While only three of the thirty-five patients whose treatment was limited at Outerboro survived to discharge from the hospital, seven of thirty-two did so at Countryside. Some of these cases, however, can be explained either as the result of patient, rather than physician, preference or as artifacts of the discharge process:

Of the three cases at Outerboro, two were cases in which treatment was withheld at the insistence of the patient and over the strenuous objections of the ICU physicians, based precisely on the perception that neither patient was dying and therefore not an appropriate candidate for limiting treatment. The third case was that of a woman with cancer who was discharged from the hospital to a nursing home, only to return quickly to the hospital, where she died less than three weeks after her discharge.

Of the seven cases at Countryside, one involved a patient whose family insisted on a transfer to another hospital. Although I was not able to follow her case to the second hospital, it is likely that she died there. A second was a patient who had refused intubation on her admission to the ICU. She was described to me as "a rare commodity . . . a patient who makes a decision on her own."

Yet, after these anomalous cases are excluded, the difference is even more striking. There are no cases at Outerboro in which physicians, of their own volition, limited treatment for a patient who survived significantly beyond a hospital discharge. At Countryside there are five: four patients who survived to hospital discharge albeit without any resolution of their underlying conditions (AIDS in one case, severe chronic respiratory disease in two others, and severe heart disease in the fourth) and a fifth who represented a technical mistake (a woman in sepsis whose DNR order was rescinded when she did far better than any of the physicians had expected). At both hospitals the principle is the same. Limit treatment only for patients who are terminal. But the application—and the meaning of "terminal"—is significantly different.

In summary, the physicians at Outerboro and Countryside make similar distinctions in determining whether a patient's medical condition warrants limiting treatment. At both hospitals, physicians advocate limiting treatment for patients who are terminal. At both hospitals, physicians are likelier to advocate limiting treatment for patients later in the course of disease rather than earlier. Moreover, at neither hospital do physicians engage, at least blatantly, in any of the types of discrimination of which they are sometimes accused: discrimination on the basis of age, on the basis of "social worth," or even, aside from judgments about the possibility of regaining consciousness, on the basis of quality of life.

At least on the surface, physicians limit themselves to technical discriminations, between patients who are incurable and those who are not. Yet these discriminations also allow for considerable latitude. To be sure, most discussions of limiting treatment take the form of technical questions. Is a patient, in fact, incurable? What is the natural history of a disease? What are the possibilities of regaining consciousness? The form allows physicians to think that they are not engaged in a process of value judgment. But form, at least in this instance, does not dictate content, and value judgment is perhaps inevitable. "Terminal," in particular, may mean terminal in the shorter run— or in the longer run. Thus, buried in technical discussions are deep and largely unarticulated differences in general orientations. Physicians are more cautious about limiting treatment at Outerboro, less so at Countryside. Although the principles are the same, the application is different. In this difference—masked by the language of prognosis and diagnosis, by the results of laboratory tests and probability estimates—is the open moral space of American medicine. It is a space quickly filled with physicians' values.

Withholding, Withdrawing, and Aggressive Treatment

While the concept of a "terminal" patient is used by physicians to extend their own discretion, a distinction between withholding and withdrawing treatment would seem to express the limits of that discretion. Because of prohibitions imposed by the law and by hospital administrators, physicians do not withdraw some of the very treatments they willingly withhold. But just as the ambiguity of the concept "terminal" leaves room for physicians to insert judgments of their own, so, too, do physicians find a way to reassert discretion in the face of these prohibitions.

Not only do the physicians at Countryside limit treatment more frequently than do those at Outerboro; they do so more decisively. Most important, as I noted above, the Countryside physicians withdraw treatment as well as withhold treatment. In twelve of twenty-two unit deaths, they performed a terminal wean, turning down or turning off the respirator for incurable, respirator-dependent patients, in effect allowing them to die, usually in a matter of hours. In contrast, while they do routinely make patients DNR and withhold treatment, the Outerboro physicians do not easily withdraw treatment.

In particular, they do not discontinue respirator support, once begun, unless they believe the patient able to survive without it.

The distinction between withholding and withdrawing treatment is one that most philosophers find wanting.[7] As a number of philosophers have argued, the distinction assumes a continuity in some treatments that is not a matter of sound logical argument. Each beat of a respirator, they argue, each drop of an antibiotic could as easily be conceived as a separate treatment as it could a single, continuous treatment. They argue, for example, that taking a patient off a respirator (withdrawing treatment in the conventional distinction) is, in principle, no different from not placing a patient on a respirator in the first place (withholding). Moreover, many philosophers have argued that whatever justifies not starting a treatment in the first place would also justify stopping that treatment after it has begun.

These observations notwithstanding, many physicians nonetheless cling to a distinction between withholding and withdrawing. Thus, one Outerboro resident, who had no qualms about withholding respirator support in certain circumstances, explained that he thought taking a patient off a respirator was different:

I think a respirator is a life-saving device. There is no doubt that, if you withdraw someone who can't live [without] a respirator, you extubate them, they're going to die. There's no doubt that someone that has a blood pressure of twenty without pressors is going to die. I mean, there's no question about that and the cause and effect is quick and rapid.

The distinction between withholding and withdrawing is made not only at Outerboro. At Countryside, an intern and a nurse made similar observations during a discussion of Mr. Charles, whose case I discussed in the previous chapter.

After the ICU staff had agreed that Mr. Charles was end stage and that he should be made DNR, the discussion turned to whether or not he should be offered a terminal wean. The intern demurred: "I couldn't see just extubating this guy. . . . I don't think I could just extubate this guy and watch him not breathe." With perhaps a hint of sarcasm, John followed up: "You'd rather put him on the floor for four months?" And, turning to Mr. Charles's nurse, he asked, "Would you be comfortable with it [discontinuing respirator support]?" But the nurse answered, "I'm never comfortable with it." John persisted, explaining that he had taken patients off respirators: "It only takes a little medicine." The intern, half joking: "I'd take a little Valium, too." John: "That's how you do it, a little for the patient, a little for you." Although Mr. Charles was made

7. See, for example, Robert Veatch, *Death, Dying and the Biological Revolution* (New Haven: Yale University Press, 1976), chap. 3; Paul Ramsey, *Ethics at the Edge of Life* (New Haven: Yale University Press, 1978), chap. 4.

DNR that afternoon, he was not extubated. When he was transferred to the floor four days later, he was still on a respirator.

Neither the Outerboro resident nor the Countryside intern was making an argument firmly grounded in any ethical system. Rather, the distinction between withholding and withdrawing treatment, as it is made by physicians, derives in large part from psychological considerations. Both the Outerboro resident and the Countryside intern were primarily concerned with the transparency of the relationship between their actions and the death of a patient. Both understood that their actions would not, in fact, cause a death. That was already foreordained by the course of disease itself. Yet both wanted to avoid a situation in which they might experience their actions as a cause of death. "I think it's just very unpleasant," another resident explained,

for the physician to have that feeling of being directly responsible, immediately responsible for somebody's death. . . . A course of passive neglect is much more tolerable. I don't think it matters. I think usually the patient is going to die in a short time anyway. . . . The difference may not be significant, but it's just . . . more aesthetic.

In this sense, the distinction between withholding and withdrawing represents an attempt to escape, at least emotionally, from a grim responsibility.

Some physicians are prepared to face this responsibility. John, for example, while recognizing that there might be "practical" difficulties in withdrawing treatment of a sort that are absent in withholding treatment, insisted that he, himself, found it much easier "to start something and see how they respond. . . . I'm willing to say that I'll stop it if there's no response." An intern added:

Once you make the decision not to treat someone . . . you come to the realization that this is probably this [person's] terminal event and you shouldn't really worry about it. If you made the decision to extubate somebody, do a terminal wean, you don't do it slowly. What's the point? You made the decision. . . . You're not going to treat this person anymore, and you want to take the tube out for the purposes of them dying. Why do it over the course of twelve hours and let them die slowly . . . ? I just take the tube out. . . . It's like making a decision to go to Boston [and] then driving [around] western Mass. for three days.

Indeed, many physicians—at Outerboro as well as Countryside—themselves recognize that the distinction between withholding and withdrawing is a flimsy one. As one Outerboro resident acknowledged: "We get into this ridiculous situation where we can't take the feeding tube out but we don't transfuse him when his crit [slang for hematocrit, a measure of blood loss] is sixteen. I mean, it's ridiculous."

The difference between the two hospitals cannot, then, be explained by differences in the moral or ethical orientations of the physicians who work there. Even if there were differences in those orientations—and I have no evidence that there are—they would not explain the complete absence of terminal weans at Outerboro. Rather, the distinction between withholding and withdrawing treatment, whatever its resonance to some physicians, is imposed on physicians primarily from outside their own culture. In particular, it is imposed by the law or, more accurately (especially in the case of Outerboro), by the hospital administration's interpretation of the law. Thus, at Outerboro, unit policy forbids removing respirator-dependent patients from respirators not because it is wrong but because the hospital lawyer has declared that terminal weans are, if not illegal, at least legally questionable.[8] Thus:

In a discussion of a dying patient whose family was prepared to stop treatments, one of the residents asked: "Can we take her off the respirator if she's breathing?" Another was more assertive: "If the family agrees, can't we take her off the respirator?" But the attending held them back: "It hasn't been done in this state and, as our lawyer says, we don't want the law made here."

As a result, the Outerboro physicians insist on maintaining ventilator support even in situations in which no one—physician, patient, or family—believes it to be in the patient's best interest. In one instance, they even insisted on maintaining ventilator support even though the initiation of that treatment had clearly been a mistake.

Mrs. Williams, a 71-year-old woman with incurable lung cancer, suffered a respiratory arrest. Although Mrs. Williams's sister and her private physician had already decided that Mrs. Williams should not be resuscitated in the event of an arrest (Mrs. Williams was no longer able to participate in such discussions herself), a nurse mistakenly began to resuscitate her. Although the mistake was quickly discovered, the resuscitation effort continued and Mrs. Williams was intubated, placed on a respirator, and transferred to the ICU. When I asked one of the residents why she had been

---

8. What the law requires, in fact, is a somewhat different matter. Although New York state law did permit withholding but not withdrawing artificial nutrition and hydration throughout the course of most of my research at Outerboro, it made no such distinction in regard to ventilator support. As the New York State Task Force on Life and the Law has noted in its report *Life Sustaining Treatment: Making Decisions and Appointing a Health Care Agent* (New York: New York State Task Force on Life and the Law, 1987) p. 11, "Many health care professionals believe that there is a clear legal distinction between the withdrawal and withholding of life-sustaining treatment such as artificial respiration. There is, in fact, no support for the distinction under New York State law." Why physicians consistently misinterpret the law is a question I return to in the next chapter.

transferred to the unit when such a transfer met no one's wishes, he explained simply: "She got intubated. Once they put it in, they can't pull it."

Similar considerations apply at Countryside, although in a narrower range of circumstances. Although Massachusetts law does allow discontinuation of respirator support from dying, respirator-dependent patients, it imposes other restrictions. In particular, Massachusetts law proscribes withdrawing (although not withholding) both hydration and feeding tubes, and this proscription is honored at Countryside.

Above all, then, the distinction between withholding and withdrawing treatment expresses the limits of the physician's discretion. Having begun some treatments, they are trapped—especially at Outerboro—by a prohibition on withdrawing them. Yet to leave matters thus would be far too simple. Having had prohibitions on withdrawing imposed on them, physicians also attempt to recapture their freedom of action.

Most important, physicians attempt to recapture their freedom of action with a distinction between more and less "aggressive" treatment. In general, physicians rank cardiopulmonary resuscitation, intubation, vasopressors, and surgery as all highly aggressive treatments. Dialysis and blood transfusions occupy an intermediate point. Antibiotics and diagnostic interventions—drawing bloods for laboratory analysis, taking X-rays, placing lines for monitoring purposes—are generally ranked among the least aggressive. Having defined some treatments as more aggressive, physicians are inclined to withhold them more quickly than less aggressive ones. And they justify this inclination in terms of the patient's best interest. The very word "aggressive" implies hostility and is thus something to be avoided.

Running through the ranking of more or less aggressive treatments are a number of dimensions. Physicians see some treatments as more aggressive because they are more invasive; others, because they are out of the ordinary rather than routine; yet others, because they are riskier. Yet all of these distinctions break down at various points. Vasopressors, for example, are less invasive than the lines used to monitor cardiac output, at least in the sense that they are less painful to the patient. Still, vasopressors are usually considered more aggressive. At least in the context of an ICU, dialysis is less routine than intubation. Still, intubation is seen as more aggressive. Some of these exceptions resist explanation. Many of the exceptions, however, can be explained by one additional distinction. Physicians think of those treatments they cannot withdraw as more aggressive than those they can withdraw.

For example, on a number of occasions the Outerboro physicians were prepared to withhold vasopressors before withholding dialysis, a ranking that by other criteria makes little sense.

After rounds, I asked Steve, one of the residents, why they had decided to provide Miss Green with dialysis but withhold pressors. He told me that, in a way, the logic escaped him but that, at the same time, he understood it. The way it made sense to him is that dialysis is a discrete treatment, that Miss Green's kidney failure was reversible and that with two or three runs she might be all right. In contrast, if she got on dopamine [a type of vasopressor], she might never get off.

Similarly, cardiopulmonary resuscitation is aggressive because it implies intubation and intubation is aggressive—at least at Outerboro—because, once begun, it cannot be stopped. In contrast, dialysis and blood transfusions, which consist of unambiguously discrete treatments, become less aggressive because they do not commit the physicians to anything more than a single treatment.

At Countryside, too, ICU physicians prefer to avoid intubation of patients they believe will become respirator dependent. It is easier, at least psychologically, to keep the patient off a respirator in the first place than to remove it later. But the costs of intubation are not so great as at Outerboro. Because physicians can discontinue ventilator support at Countryside, as they cannot at Outerboro, intubation becomes less aggressive. By the same principle, feeding tubes and hydration—by most criteria part of basic, supportive care—become aggressive. As Ken explained in the case of a ventilator-dependent patient receiving dialysis, "I didn't want to put in the feeding tube because I didn't want to get into the legal thing. Once you start a feeding tube in this state, you can't withdraw it."

Physicians avoid beginning those treatments they believe the law proscribes them from withdrawing. By assimilating the distinction between those treatments they cannot withdraw and those they can into a more general distinction between more and less aggressive treatment, they justify their avoidance in terms of the patient's best interest. But unlike a distinction between more or less aggressive treatment based on degrees of invasiveness or risk of treatments, a distinction based on the ability to withdraw treatment does not speak so clearly to the patient's best interest as to the physician's freedom of action. Thus, while prohibitions on withdrawing treatment limit the physicians' discretion, their use of the concept of "aggressive" treatment helps restore it.

11

Ethics, Families, and Technical Reason

It is not only uncertainty that limits the discretion of physicians. It is also patients and their families. Indeed, many ethicists may find my persistent concentration on physicians troubling. To be sure, it is interesting to know how doctors think about decisions to limit treatment and what the consequences of those decisions are for them. But the great weight of contemporary opinion falls on the side that so basic a decision as whether or not to treat should ultimately belong to the patient or (the Cruzan decision notwithstanding), in the event that the patient is incapacitated, to those intimates best able to speak for the patient. The findings of the President's Commission for the Study of Ethical Problems in Medicine and Biomedical and Behavioral Research are, in this respect, altogether representative First, the President's Commission is entirely clear that the "final authority" for decisions to withhold treatment is the patient's:

Respect for the self-determination of competent patients is of special importance in decisions to forego life-sustaining treatment because different people will have markedly different needs and concerns during the final period of their lives. . . . A process of collaborating and sharing information and responsibility between care givers and patients generally results in mutually satisfactory decisions. Even when it does not, the primacy of a patient's interests in self-determination and honoring the patient's own view of well-being warrant leaving with the patient the final authority to decide.[1]

Second, acknowledging that many dying patients are no longer able to make decisions for themselves, the President's Commission recognized that surrogates, preferably intimates, may have to make decisions on behalf of such patients. However, even in these circumstances, the surrogate's decision should not represent his or her own wishes, but a "substituted judgment" for the patient.

1. President's Commission for the Study of Ethical Problems in Medicine and Biomedical and Behavioral Research, *Making Health Care Decisions*, vol. 1: *Report* (Washington, DC: Government Printing Office, 1982), p. 44.

Ordinarily this will be the patient's next of kin, although it may be a close friend or another relative if the responsible health care professional judges that this other person is in fact the best advocate for the patient's interests. . . . The substituted judgment standard requires that a surrogate attempt to reach the decision that the incapacitated person would make if he or she were able to choose.[2]

We could, of course, follow both the President's Commission and various other commentators through a long series of qualifications and specifications. But in this context it is not necessary. The basic point is clear. A decision to withhold treatment, whether made by the patient or by a surrogate, should represent the wishes of that patient.

There is considerable evidence that physicians endorse this basic point, at least in principle. In, for example, a national sample of physicians conducted by the Harris organization, 70 percent answered that they would be "very unlikely" to withhold cardiopulmonary resuscitation from a patient "in great pain in the end stages of a degenerative disease" so long as that patient requested that the physician "do everything . . . to maintain her life." Only 9 percent said that they were "very likely" to withhold resuscitation against the patient's wishes.[3] Similarly, over two-thirds of the physicians answered that a choice between "aggressive" and "supportive" therapy should be made jointly by the doctor and the patient; roughly a quarter answered that the decision should be the patient's alone; less than one-tenth answered that the decision should be the doctor's.[4]

The physicians at Outerboro and Countryside are in general accord as well. One Outerboro resident spoke for the majority of the staff, virtually restating the recommendations of the President's Commission:

I think it's completely up to the patient. And if the patient is mentally together, then I don't care what the family thinks. I don't think it matters what the doctor thinks either. If the patient can't make that kind of a decision, then it's the family's choice, which is always difficult because there are so many people involved. The doctor's role is to educate, is to tell them. I tell people what I would do in the same situation or what my personal feeling is. I make it clear that it's my personal feeling and that the choice is theirs.

2. Ibid., pp. 126–27, 132.
3. Louis Harris and Associates, "Views of Informed Consent and Decisionmaking: Parallel Surveys of Physicians and the Public," in President's Commission for the Study of Ethical Problems in Medicine and Biomedical and Behavioral Research, *Making Health Care Decisions*, vol. 2: *Appendices, Empirical Studies of Informed Consent* (Washington, DC: Government Printing Office, 1982), p. 251.
4. Ibid., p. 248.

Many Countryside physicians expressed similar sentiments:

People are entitled to live their lives the way they want to and die the way that they want. I wouldn't want somebody not to have therapy if it's important [to the patient]. By the same token I wouldn't want to force somebody into having therapy that they don't want. . . . My job is to try to present families with the objective data and let them make the decision as to how far we go. . . . I feel very strongly that people or people's families are entitled to make decisions about their treatment.

Not only in interviews but also on rounds, many of the attending physicians are careful to remind the staff of the priority of the patient's wishes or, in the absence of a competent patient, the family's wishes on behalf of the patient. Just as they routinely review the hemodynamics or fluid balances of critically ill patients, equally routinely do physicians review the state of the patient's or family's wishes. "What did Mr. X. want?" "What does the wife think?" "What does the son say?"

All of this is impressive. It is also deceptive.

Physicians' acceptance of patients' or families' wishes, in principle, masks a far more complex reality in practice. When patients or families want to limit treatment in cases of incurable illness, physicians are usually (although not always) sympathetic. But this is easily explained by physicians' more general preference for treating incurable patients unaggressively. However, when a patient or family wants "everything" done, physicians are often bitterly resentful. To be sure, in some instances, physicians will honor wishes to treat incurable patients aggressively, even when they personally hold reservations. More often, though, in these circumstances, physicians resist, searching for grounds to justify limiting treatment despite the wishes of patients and families.

In stressing physicians' resistance to the wishes of patients and families, I do not question the sincerity with which they accept patients' legitimate priority in matters bearing on values. Physicians do not typically defend their discretion by claiming explicit jurisdiction over such matters. Indeed, physicians rarely question the values of their patients, regardless of whether those values are embedded in a fully articulated religious system with a specific doctrine bearing on medical treatment (as is the case among both Jehovah's Witnesses and Orthodox Jews) or are simply part of a loose set of orientations and predilections. Rather, when physicians do resist the wishes of patients and their families, they justify that resistance by moving decisions from the realm of values to the realm of technique. Thus, physicians argue, frequently and insistently, that some decisions are not value laden at all but simply technical. As such, many physicians argue, they are beyond the proper range not only of patients and families but of both the law and ethics more generally.

This is not to say that physicians always agree among themselves. Some physicians are inclined to see the proper reach of values as broader, granting greater discretion to families. Others are inclined to see the proper reach of technical considerations as broader, claiming greater jurisdiction for themselves. As a result, there are frequent disagreements whether to honor a patient's or family's wishes. But the resolution of these disagreements rarely turns on a question of ethics in a narrow sense. The doctors at Outerboro and Countryside do not show much taste for the kind of arguments that animate much of contemporary medical ethics. They are not likely, for example, to discuss the relative benefits of autonomy and benevolence or to draw fine distinctions among different procedural safeguards of a patient's rights. Rather, doctors' disagreements typically turn on the relative importance they attach to technical considerations rather than ethical considerations of any sort.

Neither is it to say that, when they do resist, physicians are always successful. Sometimes patients and families get their way despite objections. My first concern, however, is to explain how physicians justify their resistance to the wishes of patients and families and how they justify that resistance both to families and, more important, to themselves. Only after I have described what amount to the physicians' ideological tools of the trade will I return, through the vehicle of two extended case studies, to a discussion of the conditions under which physicians resist successfully and those in which they do not.

Although there is some danger of overstating the differences between the two units, the Outerboro physicians are somewhat more likely to resist families by discounting their wishes. In contrast, the Countryside physicians, while somewhat more sympathetic to the wishes of families, have also developed more explicit justifications (and procedures) for reserving certain decisions to themselves.

From Ethics to Medicine

Differences in emphasis notwithstanding, physicians at both hospitals justify their resistance to patients' and families' wishes in a number of ways.

1. *Shaping the patient's wishes.* First, a caveat: the notion that physicians resist patients' wishes assumes that patients have well-formed and well-

articulated wishes. Some do. An occasional patient will have a "living will," a written statement providing directions for care at the end of life. Others will have had explicit discussions with families and friends. But most do not or have not. As a result, families or friends, called on to act as surrogates for impaired patients, are unlikely to know what the patient would have wanted. Moreover, many patients and families enter the intensive care unit with a considerable reservoir of goodwill toward physicians, prepared to rely on their judgments and to trust their recommendations. As a result, many families are prepared, from the very beginning, to go along with whatever physicians recommend.

Mrs. Kessler was admitted to the Outerboro ICU unresponsive, with severe pneumonia and an obstructive endotracheal mass. On rounds, the morning after her admission, an intern reported that he had spoken to Mrs. Kessler's son: "I talked to the family last night. Really all I got from them was thanks for calling and that's all. . . . I talked about code status. I got to the point of asking what to do if her heart stopped, and he said, 'I guess you've got to do what you've got to do.'" Left to their own discretion by the son's Sphinx-like declaration, the ICU staff decided to make Mrs. Kessler a DNR but to treat her aggressively in other respects.

Even when families are more involved than Mrs. Kessler's, physicians rarely take their wishes as given. Physicians do not simply respond to families' requests for guidance. They actively seek out that role.

During a discussion of whether or not to dialyze Mrs. Green, a 71-year-old woman, unresponsive and with leukemia, one of the Outerboro interns explained that he had not discussed dialysis with "the family." A resident suggested that a discussion with Mrs. Green's surrogates was premature: "First, we have to decide what we want to do. . . . It depends on how we present it." An attending agreed: "The family will do what we want."

During a discussion of Mr. Greenwell, an 84-year-old who had been admitted to the Countryside ICU for severe pulmonary edema, an intern explained that Greenwell had been intubated at the urging of his private physician. "The problem," Ken said of Greenwell's wife, "is that she's hearing different things from different people. You can convince families about doing anything you want if you have strong convictions."

Although decisions to limit treatment are, for physicians, almost routine, they are hardly so for patients and families. Families, in particular, rely on physicians not only for estimates of a patient's "chances," but also for explanations of unfamiliar procedures and perhaps even for a diffuse sense of what constitutes "appropriate" medical care. The technological complexity of intensive care medicine—with constant monitoring, diagnostic tests, and the often intimidating sight of respirators and lines—only increases the dependence of families on physicians. As a result, as one Outerboro resident,

Karen, explained, physicians' recommendations are usually sufficient to convince a patient's family that "enough is enough:"

Most families don't want to know the gory details of what you would do to these patients if you didn't let them die. . . . I think the doctor has to assess the likelihood of this person surviving and what kind of life they're going to have if they survive. And then, with that thought, bring up to the family what the doctor has decided. Then, if the family has strong objections, then you take them into consideration. I find that most families, if you really made a medically sound decision about whether or not they should have extensive measures taken, most families will agree that enough is enough.

Often advice is disguised in the form of a question. But as a second resident pointed out, a good deal depends on the way physicians pose that question:

We say, you know, when we try to convince someone to make a patient Do Not Resuscitate, we'll say, "Do you want us to pump on his chest?" That doesn't terrify them. "Sure, doctor." But they don't understand the full implications of that. "Do you want us put him on a breathing machine, you know, and keep him alive even when the rest of him is dead?" and they understand that quite well.

Physicians also enjoy considerable latitude in their selection of a surrogate. Families are rarely of a single mind. Friends without ties to the patient of either blood or marriage—a category of considerable importance both on account of high divorce rates and because of the increasing presence in the ICU of gay men with AIDS—may make claims, separate from a conventional family's, to decide for the patient. The jumble of family life gives physicians a choice. "What we usually ask," an attending explained to a resident troubled by the persistent intrusions of one woman on behalf of a comatose friend, "is for the family to appoint a representative. . . . I'd like to get her off the front line. She's not family." By picking and choosing (albeit within a limited range) among potential surrogates, the Outerboro and Countryside physicians are able to increase the likelihood of finding one who will abide by their recommendations.

Most often, then, physicians do not have to resist the wishes of patients or their families, because physicians themselves have shaped those wishes. But even when the patient or, more often, the patient's family persists in asking for a course of treatment, the ICU physician is equipped with a large number of techniques for discounting those wishes.

2. *Discounting the family: Emotional considerations.* Even when a family persists, its wishes may be either ignored or discounted on the somewhat curious ground that they are emotionally too involved in the case. This takes two forms, both more in evidence at Outerboro than at Countryside.

First, physicians may use the emotional involvement of the family as a justification for shielding the family from involvement in difficult decisions. As Karen, whose comments I cited in the previous section, continued:

Most families don't want that decision. They want you to tell them what you think is best. I mean, that can be abused. I guess you can make the wrong decision. But I don't think it's right to give families that guilt, to decide whether or not, you know, 'cause they take it as guilt. Well, I told them not to do anything: It's my fault.

Similar sentiments were echoed frequently on rounds at Outerboro: "You can't let him make that decision. He's got to live with it for the rest of his life"; "I think the daughter knows she's not doing well. . . . We all agree the family shouldn't have to be in the position of having to say maybe a little more hemo[dialysis]." Although there is certainly considerable good faith in these observations, they also serve an ideological purpose. They make it unnecessary even to attempt to shape the family's wishes. Those wishes may be ignored (or assumed) altogether and without discussion, all in the name of what is presented as the family's own good.

Second, by focusing on the emotional involvement of the family, ICU physicians may turn the family itself into an object of treatment. At one point in a discussion of an incurably ill 73-year-old man, an Outerboro attending suggested, "You have to diagnose the family. You get angries, deniers, accepters." Such formulations are expressions of sympathy for the excruciatingly difficult process of watching the prolonged death of a friend, a father, mother, husband, or wife. But they also serve to discount the family's wishes. "You're going into psychiatry," Dennis, an Outerboro attending, said to an intern during a discussion of a 70-year-old woman who had just suffered a severe heart attack and stroke. "What do you make of the son? He's very unstable." Conceptualizing the family as an object of treatment subtly shifts the emphasis from thinking of the family as an active agent in medical decisions, with rights at least coequal to those of physicians, to thinking of the family as something to be acted upon.

In either form, an emphasis on the family's emotional involvement helps the Outerboro physicians justify the sway of their own inclinations in decisions to limit treatment.

3. *Discounting wishes: Technical considerations.* If some wishes can be discounted because family or friends are emotionally too involved, others can be discounted because they lack sufficient technical information. As one Countryside resident complained, "They watch television. They want someone to say they have two weeks," without understanding the limits of medical prognostics. An Outerboro resident made the same point more generally:

A lot of times we approach them and say . . . "Would you like us to do everything for the patient, or would you like us to make him comfortable?" I think that under very rare circumstances is the family able to make that decision. They've never worked in an ICU. They've never worked in a hospital. They don't know the prognosis. They don't have any idea what goes on in an ICU. I think . . . their opinions are given far too much weight.

To be sure, there are occasional exceptions, families or friends who do know "what goes on in an ICU" or who have "worked in a hospital." Thus, when the mother-in-law of a unit secretary was admitted to the Countryside ICU, the unit physicians looked to her to provide leadership for the rest of her family. Similarly, an Outerboro resident, Steve, recalled: "Sometimes you see, like with Mr. Finkel, the daughter was a psychiatrist or a psychologist who was very familiar with . . . medicine and with the ethical issues of prolonging life." But these are exceptions that prove the more general rule. Before surrogates can make decisions on behalf of dying patients, the physicians at both Outerboro and Countryside believe, those surrogates must possess some knowledge of medical procedures. Even the expression of values in these formulations depends on technical knowledge. And with few exceptions only physicians possess that knowledge.

The claim that a dense knowledge of medical procedures is a requisite to sound decisions can be used to discount not only the expressed wishes of a surrogate but also those of the patient himself or herself. This is particularly the case when those wishes were expressed before admission to the unit:

Mrs. Rosen, a 35-year-old woman with advanced metastatic cancer and now minimally responsive, had earlier expressed a wish for aggressive treatment. She had, one Outerboro intern reported, wanted "everything" done. A resident pointed out that she was "up and driving around until she came in." But another resident, chafing at the continued treatment of an incurable patient, argued: "I don't think she knew what was in store for her. I don't think anyone can know unless he's a physician."

Whether or not to limit treatment comes to depend, at least in the physician's formulation, on medical knowledge. An ethical issue becomes a technical one.

4. *Quality of life as a technical concern.* Of all the issues relevant to withholding treatment, the most difficult for physicians to claim as their own are those bearing on what kind of life is worth living, on what is usually called "quality of life." Especially at Outerboro, physicians—predominantly white, heavily upper middle class in origin and uniformly upper middle class in destination—are ill-equipped to make judgments about what may be, in the language of the President's Commission, the "markedly different needs and

concerns" of a patient population that is heavily black, Hispanic, and poor. To be sure, the physicians at both Outerboro and Countryside are often concerned about the quality of life available to patients after leaving the unit. Similarly, they acknowledge the right of families and friends to invoke quality of life in determining what a patient would have wanted. But they assert no explicit right of their own to limit treatment on the basis of such considerations. They do not intend to consider quality of life.

Yet, despite their best intentions, a characteristic turn of language does, in some extreme cases, introduce judgments about quality of life.

On a "minimally responsive" man with metastatic cancer: "He had a quality of life."

On a man apparently making "purposive" motions but unresponsive to commands: "We've lost his mental status for a long time."

On an AIDS patient, unresponsive except to pain: "He has AIDS with no mental status." And later: "I didn't know him before, if he was a person."

On a 92-year-old man with metastatic cancer, unresponsive except to deep pain: "We've decided that his sister wants to keep him as a pet. We can keep his body alive."

Quality of life is fundamentally a multidimensional concept, with infinite gradations. As a result, judgments about quality of life require weighing often incomparable "needs and concerns." But if a patient has "no mental status," is not "a person," is nothing more than "a pet," then quality of life becomes something that may be altogether absent.[5] Quality of life becomes, in effect, a dichotomy. Whether there is *any* "quality of life" becomes a technical judgment appropriately made by physicians.

5. *Narrowing the scope of decisions.* On very general mandates to treat aggressively or, in the most frequent formulation, to "do everything," physicians will at least affect to honor the wishes of a patient or a family. However, decisions to withhold treatment are not usually made in general. They are made in specific, treatment by treatment. But if general mandates seem the proper realm of values—and, thus, of patients and families—decisions about specific treatments are in the realm of technical considerations and, thus, of doctors.

One strategy, then, that doctors pursue when confronted with a family that wants everything done is to narrow the area of decision making. When Mrs. Sanders, a woman with metastatic cancer, was admitted to the Countryside

---

5. A few of the younger doctors, although none of the attendings, will on occasion point out the value judgments implicit in these formulations. Thus, one resident argued, in the final case cited above, "Even if they want to keep him in the hospital as a pet, that's their right." Far from vitiating my general point, her comment makes it explicit.

ICU following a cardiac arrest, the resident duly noted, "Prior to the cardiac arrest, she wanted everything done," but quickly added, "whatever that means" and moved right on from a discussion of "aggressive care" in general to the specific issue of whether or not to place a Swan-Ganz catheter.

Once physicians have narrowed the scope of the decision, they are on firmer ground. If patients, or families on their behalf, have the right to set a general orientation to treatment, they do not have the right, at least according to the doctors at Outerboro and Countryside, to demand specific treatments or to pick and choose among treatments.

Mr. Dean had been admitted to the Countryside ICU from a nursing home with severe hypertension and end stage renal disease. Dean's family had said they did not want him to be treated aggressively. But they were also asking that he be kept on dialysis and be given pressors. Ken wouldn't hear of it: "Then this patient is going out. Families can't manipulate the system this way."

Mr. Edwards, a 57-year-old AIDS patient at Outerboro, had "said yes to everything." As Mr. Edwards's mental status declined over the course of a week, his sister and nephew continued to press for aggressive treatment. When it became apparent that Mr. Edwards would need dialysis, the medical staff was reluctant to provide it for a man now clearly dying. An attending suggested that "it all depends on his lungs. That's how I would make my decision." A resident added: "So it's really regardless of what the family wants."

Mark, an Outerboro attending, made the general point:

If the medical decision says it shouldn't be done, it shouldn't be done. . . . Because if you do everything the family says, then if they say give the patient a heart transplant and it just so happened that a donor was available, they'd get a heart transplant, no matter if they were 90 and irrevocably senile [with] permanent brain damage. And we don't do that as a matter of fact. They don't transplant kidneys into 90 [year olds]. So there is a limit to what we'll do.

Once the decision has become defined as a decision about a specific treatment, it becomes exclusively medical.

Not all the physicians at Outerboro or Countryside would make claims so blunt or so sweeping as Mark's. Yet nearly all would reserve some decisions to themselves. Patients and their families may provide general directives for care at the end of life. But physicians make decisions not (or not just) about "aggressive care" in general but about specific treatments. And, while they may insist on respecting the wishes of the patient in general, they may reserve decisions about specific treatments to themselves.

6. *Futility.* Underlying the strategy of narrowing the scope of decisions is a more general argument. Even when a family insists they "do everything,"

physicians may justify withholding treatment on grounds of the technical judgment that further treatment is futile. This argument is heard frequently at both Outerboro and Countryside.

The clearest and least controversial grounds on which physicians deny treatment on grounds of its futility is a determination of brain death. Although the following example is drawn from Outerboro, other similar examples could easily be drawn from Countryside as well.

Mrs. Huff, a 69-year-old woman, had suffered a severe stroke. According to an intern, her "family wasn't prepared to deal with this information." An attending asked rhetorically, "What if the family says, do everything, and we find her brain dead?" He answered his own question: "Dead is when the doctors say she's dead."

Death, in this formulation, is clearly a technical judgment. The family's wishes are entirely beside the point.

Although there is general agreement among lawmakers and ethicists that brain death is a technical judgment, physicians make similar claims in other circumstances where consensus is not so sure.[6] At Outerboro, for example, one attending argued that the ICU staff could withhold dialysis from a 66-year-old woman without the specific consent of the patient's daughter because the treatment would be "futile."

The daughter of Mrs. Simms, a 66-year-old woman with severe cardiac disease, had requested that her mother not be treated aggressively. The morning after Mrs.

---

6. See, for example, the President's Commission for the Study of Ethical Problems in Medicine and Biomedical and Behavioral Research, *Defining Death* (Washington, DC: Government Printing Office, 1981). For efforts to justify futility as grounds for discontinuing treatment, see Tom Tomlinson and Howard Brody, "Futility and the Ethics of Resuscitation," *Journal of the American Medical Association* 264 (1990): 1276–80; J. Charles Hackler and F. Charles Hiller, "Family Consent to Orders Not to Resuscitate," *Journal of the American Medical Association* 264 (1990): 1281–83. For statements critical of the concept of futility, see Stuart Youngner, "Who Defines Futility?" *Journal of the American Medical Association* 260 (1988): 2094–95; John D. Lantos, Peter A. Singer, Robert M. Walker, Gregory P. Gramelspeacher, Gary P. Shapiro, Miguel A. Sanchez-Gonzalez, Carol B. Stocking, Steven H. Miles, and Mark Siegler, "The Illusion of Futility in Clinical Practice," *American Journal of Medicine* 87 (1989): 81–84. Recent guidelines from the Council on Ethical and Judicial Affairs of the American Medical Association tilt toward the critical position but with considerable ambiguity. The guidelines state that, "in the unusual circumstance where efforts to resuscitate a patient are judged by the treating physician to be futile, *even if previously requested by the patient,* CPR may be withheld." But this statement follows a criticism of the ways in which some physicians determine futility and an insistence on a definition of futility that "respects the autonomy and value judgments of individual patients" and is based on the patient's determination of "what is or is not of benefit, in keeping with his or her personal values and priorities." Council on Ethical and Judicial Affairs, American Medical Association, "Guidelines for the Appropriate Use of Do-Not-Resuscitate Orders," *Journal of the American Medical Association* 265 (1991): 1868–71.

Simms's death, an attending summarized the medical judgments of her final days. "It became very apparent she would need dialysis. Her daughter thought the patient would not want cardiopulmonary resuscitation. So we took it upon ourselves not to dialyze, which we thought would be futile."

In a second instance—during a discussion of whether to transfuse Mr. Figueroa, a 57-year-old man with incurable kidney disease, whose case I discussed briefly in chapter 9—an Outerboro attending extended the principle of futility from grounds for specifying a family's otherwise unspecified wishes to grounds for ignoring the wishes of a family altogether.

One of the residents had suggested that a transfusion would put a drain on the blood bank. The attending objected strenuously to an argument made on such grounds. However, after listing a number of reasons why Mr. Figueroa could not recover, he did suggest that a decision to withhold blood could be made on other grounds that were "out of the family's hands": "Mrs. Shabazz's family [a reference to a patient who had recently died] could have refused to write a consent form for her to die and she still would have died. . . . It's nicer to have the family along because it avoids some discomfort. That's where the social factors come in."

In yet another case—a comatose man dying of AIDS, whose sister was nonetheless insisting that he be resuscitated in the event of an arrest—the same attending extended the argument. During morning rounds he suggested that, while the patient could not be made DNR, he was "CNR," "Can Not Resuscitate," thus removing the question of resuscitation from the moral authority of the family to the technical judgment of physicians.

At Outerboro the transformation of patients' wishes to technical issues is explicit. At Countryside the transformation not only is equally explicit but takes on a collective character, as semiofficial policy, lacking at Outerboro. Indeed, the bluntest formulation of the technical basis for decision making was expressed not by a physician but by a Countryside administrator and member of that hospital's Ethics Committee: "No one," she said, "has a right to a treatment that's futile." Moreover, an appeal to the futility of a treatment as grounds for denying that treatment is invoked in a wider range of circumstances at Countryside than at Outerboro. In particular, while the Outerboro physicians rarely, if ever, claim the right to issue a Do Not Resuscitate order in the face of a family's objections, the Countryside physicians do.

The Countryside ICU staff was considering whether or not to write a Do Not Resuscitate order for Mr. Lake, a 73-year-old man who had been admitted to the unit with acute renal failure, a gastrointestinal bleed, pneumonia, and sepsis. Ken asked what they should do "if the family wanted a full court press." One of the residents started to say what he thought were the "interesting ethical issues." But Ken cut him off, arguing that the decision depended entirely on prognostics: "There are no ethical issues. . . . I'm not an ethicist. I'm a doctor." When the resident attempted to distinguish different circumstances preceding codes, Ken broke in again: "A code is a code. It's a medical decision, not an ethical decision."

In the case of Mrs. Diaz, a 79-year-old woman with metastatic cancer, a Countryside resident argued for a "unilateral decision" against CPR, resisting the expressed wishes not just of a family but of a competent patient herself. The case is also remarkable because the resident was willing to state his argument not just in the relatively private setting of rounds but also in a medical chart, subject to public review.

Pt last noc [night] expressed to RN "I want to die." When I spoke [with] her this AM she expressed the same, adding "my life is miserable." However, when asked about whether or not she would want her heart "shocked" to "restart it" if it should stop, chest compressions or reintubation she replied "I suppose so." Again informed of diagnosis of lung CA [cancer] which she stated she was unaware of despite documentation in chart that she has been told of this. Informed of probable futility of CPR in light of underlying problems. I do not believe that CPR should be performed on this pt regardless of her expressed thoughts as it will not significantly change her outcome/prognosis and is not medically indicated. I feel that unilateral decision should be made not to perform CPR but will defer this to her attending of record, Dr. Novak (although I would be willing to write the note and accept responsibility).

Although the argument is made in a broader range of circumstances at Countryside than at Outerboro, the underlying logic is the same at both. The technical judgment that a treatment is futile becomes the basis for a decision to withhold treatment. But a technical judgment raises no issues of values and requires no consultation with family or friends. Ethics is transformed into medicine.

Decision Making as Negotiation

Whether physicians are justified in extending the claims of technical reason, I do not presume to judge. While some ethicists or philosophers might defend the physicians' claims and others contest them, it is enough for my purposes to note that the boundaries between the technical and the ethical are, at least in part, social constructions. They are social constructions because technical judgments, as I suggested earlier, are inherently probabilistic. The determination that a 1 percent chance or a one-tenth of 1 percent chance of success, another day or another hour of life amounts to "futility" depends not on logic but on social convention. Even more fundamentally, they are social constructions because they are contested and because their acceptance in practice (if not their logical or analytic validity) depends in part on the skill, assertiveness, and social position of those who make claims. Whatever the truth of the matter in a more philosophical sense, physicians' claims for the domain of the technical are, at the very least, convenient, for they allow physicians to reconcile two otherwise irreconcilable values. They allow physicians to acknowledge the rights of patients in matters of values while, at the same time, preserving their own ability to make decisions. This is no small accomplishment.

All this, however, takes place in the realm of ideology. I have cited physicians discussing termination of treatment with each other during rounds, with an interviewer, and, in one instance, through a note in a chart. They are talking about patients and their families. But they are not talking to those patients or families so much as to themselves. They are attempting to convince themselves of their own rights. They do not always succeed. Among the cases just cited, Mr. Figueroa was, as noted earlier, in fact provided with transfusions at the insistence of both his family and a consulting physician. In the case of Mr. Lake, the Countryside physicians themselves eventually decided that a Do Not Resuscitate order was not warranted. And in the case of Mrs. Diaz, her "attending of record" decided against withholding treatment. Still, the ICU physicians are not simply posturing when they assert their right to make unilateral decisions. If they do not always succeed in convincing themselves to go ahead with unilateral decisions, they succeed sometimes and in bits and pieces.

To say with any precision how often physicians make decisions to terminate treatment and how often patients or their families do so is impossible. I can find several cases at both Outerboro and Countryside in which physicians did withhold some treatment against the expressed wishes of patients or their families, and several others in which they withheld treatment in the absence of expressed wishes. But any effort to provide an exact count would be both an understatement and an overstatement. It would be an understatement because it would leave out those instances in which physicians simply did not offer a treatment which, if offered, a family might have pursued. It would be an overstatement because it would include instances in which physicians withheld some treatment but nonetheless accommodated the wishes of families in other respects. And, most important, any attempt to count is deceptive because it assumes that the wishes of physicians, patients, and families exist prior to a decision when in fact they often do not. Not only do physicians shape the wishes of patients and families. But so, too, do patients and families shape the preferences of physicians.

In any specific situation, a decision is the result of a complex process of negotiation and mutual adjustment. In this process, the willingness of physicians to proceed on their own or with varying degrees of agreement from patients and families depends on their judgment about the patient, the patient's condition, the character of the treatment in question, the strength of the patient's family's convictions, and the strength of their own convictions. At the same time, the degree to which a patient or family is willing to insist on doing everything depends on many of the same considerations as well as on the skill of physicians in mounting a compelling argument.

The process of negotiation cannot, however, be described fully in the abstract. Rather, it can be described only in the course of detailed analyses of concrete cases. In what follows, I draw, by way of illustration, on two such cases, one from Outerboro and one from Countryside.

The Case of Scranton Haskell

Mr. Haskell, a 73-year-old former construction worker, was admitted to Outerboro for gastrointestinal bleeding and a possible heart attack. At the time of his admission Mr. Haskell had also been undergoing evaluation as an outpatient for a mass in his lung. On the seventh day of Mr. Haskell's hospitalization, a lab report confirmed a "poorly differentiated malignant tumor . . . most likely metastatic to skin." The following day, in order to manage his continued bleeding and to monitor his hemodynamic status, Mr. Haskell was transferred to the ICU. On the ninth day of his hospitalization, his first in the ICU, one of the unit attendings, Sam, wanted to know whether Mr. Haskell and his family were aware that the diagnosis of cancer had been confirmed. Told that they were not, he suggested reservations about an unlimited course of treatment: "I think we have to sit down with the wife and discuss what we know and what we suspect, holding nothing back." However, as an intern explained the following morning, Mr. Haskell himself "doesn't want his wife to know how sick he is." The discussion with the wife was postponed. On the eleventh day of his hospitalization, Mr. Haskell was intubated and placed on a respirator.

By the twenty-second day of Mr. Haskell's hospital stay, his bleeding had slowed and the ICU staff was attempting, slowly, to wean him from the respirator. Because he was sedated and intubated, Mr. Haskell's mental status was difficult to assess. He did, however, continue to respond to commands by blinking his eyes and squeezing hands. There was no treatment available for his underlying cancer. Sam summarized the situation, expressing deference to the wishes of Mr. Haskell's family but reiterating his reservations about "aggressive" treatment:

We have continued with our aggressive support because we wanted to clear up the picture, because the patient is awake, and because the family has not approached us. Fortunately, we have not had to deal with a cardiac arrest or dialysis. I think we should be supportive of the family but make them aware this is a terminal illness. I don't think he is prepared to deal with that kind of data.

The following day, with Mr. Haskell's mental status declining, a resident reported that he had spoken to Mrs. Haskell. At the same time, he began to prepare for a decision to withhold treatment, independent of her wishes, by questioning her judgment. "I talked to the wife yesterday. She has very poor insight. Basically, she wants him kept alive." He also reported that she had liquor on her breath. Sam acknowledged Mrs. Haskell's wishes but subtly shifted the grounds for respecting them from a respect for rights to psychological and humane concerns: "We really should not try to browbeat this lady. She's going through hell." Moreover, Sam immediately qualified his acceptance of Mrs. Haskell's wishes:

But we should view dramatic interventions [cautiously]. If we have to deal with dialysis, we'll deal with that when we have to. If there's a cardiac arrest, we should institute therapy but we don't have to sustain it and we can send him to the East Wing [a "step-down" unit equipped for patients on respirators, but with less intensive nursing and medical care].

Sam's comments turned a neat trick. On the one hand, they expressed sympathy for Mrs. Haskell. On the other hand, they removed two issues—how actively to respond in the event of an arrest and where in the hospital Mr. Haskell should be treated—from the realm of Mrs. Haskell's rights. Thus, in a single formula, Sam managed both to respect and to resist Mrs. Haskell's right to decide.

The twenty-sixth day of Mr. Haskell's hospitalization was the first of the month, and two new physicians, Mark and Dennis, began their rotations as unit attendings. "The family," an intern explained, "wants absolutely everything." But neither Mark nor Dennis was prepared to accept so uncritically the family's wishes. With pointed rhetoric—"If the family wanted a heart transplant, would we give it?"—Mark suggested that some decisions are not up to the family. Dennis followed Mark's line of reasoning: "If he bleeds, do we want to transfuse?" A resident answered: "The family says yes, but we say something different." But Dennis would not accept this formulation: "No, the wife doesn't say yes." Some decisions are not the family's. Moreover, Dennis took another tack—"We have to establish a relationship with the family"—suggesting that the residents should be able to exert more influence on Mrs. Haskell's wishes. Dennis was prepared to respect the wishes of Mrs. Haskell but only if he could shape those wishes. At the same time, if he could not shape her wishes, he was searching for decisions that could be the physicians' alone.

On the twenty-ninth day of his hospital stay, Mr. Haskell had begun to bleed again. Mrs. Haskell continued to press for aggressive treatment. After rounds, an intern noted in Mr. Haskell's chart, "Plan not to tx w/ [transfuse with] blood as per grim prognosis," the first explicit order in Mr. Haskell's chart to withhold a potentially life-sustaining treatment. On the thirty-first day, the ICU staff successfully weaned Mr. Haskell from the respirator. On rounds, one of the residents asked whether to reintubate Mr. Haskell if his breathing worsened. Mark answered that they should not: "I'd put it, 'It's futile.' That means it's not a family decision. So we shouldn't ask the family if they want him back on the respirator if he worsens. We can just say it won't do anything." That afternoon, off the respirator, Mr. Haskell was transferred to a bed on the wards. Later that afternoon, apparently convinced by the transfer, Mrs. Haskell agreed to make her husband DNR. A note in Mr. Haskell's chart read simply: "Given critical nature of pts disease, and clearly poor prognosis, decision for supportive care only made by family." Mr. Haskell died three days later.

The final note cited from Haskell's chart is hardly a full account of the decision-making process. Although the Outerboro physicians were happy to assign final responsibility for the decision to withhold cardiac respiration and ventilator support to Mrs. Haskell, her agreement not only was after the fact but followed prolonged efforts to convince her of the futility of treatment. In these senses, the decision was the physicians'.

That the ICU physicians would, eventually, decide unilaterally to withhold potentially life-prolonging treatments from Mr. Haskell was almost overdetermined. Haskell had never made his own wishes clear and had excluded his wife from the decision-making process. When Haskell was no longer able to participate in decisions himself, his wife was both ill-prepared to take part and, because of her drinking, easily disqualified. Moreover, two succeeding teams of attendings had prepared the way for withholding treatment on grounds of futility. Nonetheless, they waited until the twenty-ninth day of Haskell's hospital stay and the twenty-second day of his ICU stay before finally deciding to withhold additional blood transfusions. What they would have done had Haskell arrested before that decision is a matter only for speculation. Although the final decision to withhold treatment can be attributed to Mrs. Haskell only with the most generous stretch of the imagination, it is nonetheless clear that she delayed that decision long beyond the point at which the physicians caring for her husband would have liked to have made it.

The Case Of Kelly Connors

Kelly Connors was a 20-year-old preschool teacher. She had been admitted to the Countryside Intensive Care Unit from the Emergency Room of a nearby hospital, where her parents and fiance had taken her for what they described as "flu-like" symptoms. But the physicians in the Emergency Room quickly realized that Kelly was suffering from something far more serious than the flu. They immediately transferred her to Countryside for treatment of acute renal failure complicated by bilateral pneumonia, hypoxia, and hemoptysis. Recognizing the acute character of Kelly's condition, the ICU physicians began her on emergency dialysis for her renal failure and treated her acute respiratory distress with a special, rarely used jet ventilator. Kelly made it through the night, and the next morning the unit physicians and nurses were congratulating themselves on a remarkable "save." For nearly four weeks, with her father, mother, fiance, and younger sister camped out in the waiting room, often overnight, Kelly made slow progress. As her respiration improved and her sedation lightened, she became more responsive. She was taken off the jet respirator and placed on a regular one. Although Kelly continued to need regular dialysis, Ken began to think of weaning her from the respirator. Over the course of those four weeks, many of the unit's doctors and nurses seemed to develop a genuine affection for Kelly and her family. Ken, in particular, singled Kelly out for special attention. One evening, while getting ready to leave, he instructed the housestaff, "I'm not on tonight, but for this patient . . . ," and he hit his beeper. There was no thought in his mind, in the mind of any of the housestaff or any of the many consultants who had helped with Kelly's care, of withholding any treatment from a young woman who seemed to be coming through so protracted a crisis.

I first talked to Kelly's father, Tom, two weeks into Kelly's hospital course. He was optimistic but readily admitted that Kelly's illness had been an "emotional roller coaster" for him. There could come a time, he acknowledged, when he might say "enough is enough," as his mother had once decided for his father when "we agreed . . . that we weren't going to hook [him] up." "I've even thought about it," he told me, "with Kelly. . . . If I hadn't seen any improvement, she kept getting worse and worse and worse, then you've got to start thinking seriously about it." But at the moment, "There is no decision to be made. I don't care what you have to do. You do what you have to to save her life. If you've got to cut the leg off to save her life, you are going to do it. That's the way I feel."

Late at night on the twenty-seventh day of her hospital stay, Kelly's heart stopped beating, probably a result of an infection acquired from one of the very lines used to sustain her life. Cardiopulmonary resuscitation along with heavy doses of vasopressors brought Kelly's heart back, but she was now unresponsive. As one of the interns told me the next morning, she was now "a different patient." Morning rounds at Kelly's bedside were somber. Ken admitted that he was depressed. An intern confessed that he "had always assumed she'd make it." And, in one of the strangest moments of all my research, the discussion somehow drifted to voodoo cults, the use of drugs to simulate brain death, and, finally, to zombies and the "undead"—as the ICU doctors, apparently unaware of what they were saying, dropped the guise of science to search desperately for any way of defying death.

After her arrest Kelly's condition continued to worsen. "There's not much to say medically," Ken acknowledged. "She's a train wreck. . . . Every single organ is in failure except the liver." With Kelly now unresponsive, Ken decided to press her family to make her DNR.

But Kelly's family would not agree. When I spoke to Tom two weeks after Kelly's arrest, he understood that his daughter's condition had worsened. When Ken had raised the question of making Kelly DNR, it had hit home: "He says, if she codes, how do you want to handle it? It kind of burst a lot of bubbles. . . . I'm her father. I don't want her to be this way. . . . I don't want to believe Ken. But I have relapses of what the hell happens if he's right." Where, before, Tom had often lingered in Kelly's room, now, he acknowledged, "I have a hard time staying in there with her." Still, as long as there remained any chance, he was not prepared to give up:

As long as they do an EEG [an electroencephalogram] and they see brain waves, see, I don't care how sluggish they are. She can be retrained with a lot of time, energy, effort, and love. . . . She may be a vegetable the rest of her life, and I don't know that and they don't know that. So, until they tell me she's going to be a vegetable the rest of her life, right, you are going to put out 100 percent. . . . And I'm going to fight for that right.

In face of the family's insistence, Ken was willing to express his own ambivalence: "Maybe she's coming around. I'm not trying to be overly optimistic. She's young." Ken was prepared to "keep going" but with a qualification. If Kelly woke up, Ken was even willing to put her back on the jet ventilator, but he added, "She's not awake, and I'm not going to put everyone through a week of torture with that." The new housestaff, who had rotated into the unit a week after Kelly's arrest and had never seen her when her eventual recovery seemed likely, were even less enthusiastic. "The father's bizarre," one intern claimed. "He's very accusatory of any suggestion that we're doing less than 100 percent." And the resident suggested that "there's really not much more we can do."

Three and a half weeks after her arrest, on the fifty-fourth day of her hospitalization, Kelly developed an occlusion in her lung. Ken immediately ruled out surgery as a possibility: "No one would take her." He also ruled out a special type of dual ventilation that would require reintubating Kelly: "To be honest, I'm not even going to present it to the family. We'll decide." But neither was Ken prepared to give up completely, especially given the family's wishes: "Her chances are low, but they exist. She still has a 5, 6 percent chance of a six-month recovery. In a prediction model, it's lousy. In an individual patient, it's a lot. And the family wants a full go."

An emergency bronchoscopy resolved the immediate crisis, but two days later Ken's resolve had hardened. He had talked to the family, he reported on morning rounds. "I think I finally got across to them that that's not their daughter anymore. It's not Kelly Connors any more. I'm going to be very tough with them and demand that she be made no CPR. Not withdraw care, just no CPR." If they did not agree, Ken continued, he could either withdraw from the case or, with the support of independent consultants, write a unilateral order. But when, a little later, I ran into Tom and Kelly's fiance, Jack, they were still insistent on treating Kelly as aggressively as possible. Tom could not agree to making her DNR: "It would feel like killing my own daughter," and neither he nor Jack nor his wife could go along with it. Kelly died five days later, one day short of two full months in the unit, despite the best efforts of the housestaff to resuscitate her after her final arrest.

That the Countryside physicians would treat Kelly Connors aggressively seems almost overdetermined, much as it seemed overdetermined that the Outerboro physicians would eventually withhold treatment from Scranton Haskell. Kelly was young. Her family was present almost constantly, showed no ambivalence, and acted in concert. Despite occasional efforts ("the father's bizarre"), Connors's family was harder to discount than Haskell's wife. Moreover, the Countryside physicians themselves, particularly Ken, were less certain of the eventual outcome. Given that Connors remained a full code until the very end, it would be easy to read her case as a paradigm of those situations in which families are able to insist successfully on aggressive treatment.

Still, even in the Connors case, there are ambiguities. Although Connors remained a full code, the Countryside physicians, without consulting the family, rejected the possibility of surgery when her lung occluded and on two occasions decided not to raise options of special ventilatory support.

In neither the Haskell case nor the Connors case can responsibility for a decision be assigned solely to either physicians or family. In both cases, to a greater or lesser extent, physicians considered the wishes of family. In both cases, to a greater or lesser extent, family considered the arguments of physicians. If decisions are not exactly mutual, they are at least the result of mutual influence. Moreover, even the notion of discrete decisions begins to disappear. To be sure, in both cases there are moments of high drama. But decisions are not made once and for all. With each day that Connors and Haskell remained unresponsive, the physicians' resolve to withhold treatment hardened and the families' insistence on treating aggressively weakened. Decisions were considered and reconsidered, made and remade, negotiated and renegotiated. Decisions were not an event but a process.

More generally, the picture I have drawn corresponds neither to an image of unbridled professional discretion nor to one of patients' rights triumphant. As many observers of contemporary medicine have argued, the discretion of physicians in clinical decisions (like the discretion of professionals in other fields) depends on their ability to make successful claims to the exclusive command of technical knowledge. Yet, while the physicians at Outerboro and Countryside make such claims, they do not always succeed either in convincing themselves that they are legitimate or in converting them to influence over patients and their families, for the claims of physicians are met by the counterclaims of patients and, more important, families. These counterclaims are not based fundamentally in ethics. They come, rather, from the depth of human emotions in the face of death—from hope, denial, guilt, love. There is no reason to think that families, today, would feel such emotions anymore than they have in the past or would anymore insist on "doing everything" for a wife or husband, a daughter or son. What may be different, however, is the institutionalization of patients' rights, in law and in hospital policy, in such a way as to empower families when they do insist on doing everything. In such a situation, physicians may continue to exercise considerable influence and enjoy considerable discretion. By no means have they been reduced to the role of technicians and nothing more. But at the same time, they must, at the very least, take the wishes of patients and families into account.

An alternative interpretation might subsume the empowerment of families in the rise of what some observers have called a consumer movement in medicine.[7] My point, however, is that the empowerment of families probably has less to do with a decline of trust in physicians or with more intense disagreements with them (the kind of developments emphasized by the notion of a consumer movement) than with the institutionalization of procedures and values that make existing distrust and disagreement more consequential. It is to the point, albeit anecdotally, that neither Haskell's wife nor any of Kelly Connors's family represent the young, educated, upper-middle-class patients who are usually identified as the spearhead of the consumer movement.

Is the glass half empty or half full? The answer, of course, is that it's both. From the point of view of those convinced that the rise of contemporary medical ethics has transformed the practice of medicine, the surprise is that physicians continue to exercise as much discretion as they do. From the point of view of those convinced that physicians continue to dominate patients, the surprise is that families exercise as much influence as they do. Both points of view are right.

7. See, for example, Marie R. Haug and Bebe Lavin, *Consumerism in Medicine* (Beverly Hills: Sage, 1983); Leo Reeder, "The Patient as Client-Consumer: Some Observations on the Changing Professional-Client Relationship," *Journal of Health and Social Behavior* (1972) 13: 406–12.

12

The "Do Not Resuscitate" Order as Ritual

In 1976, in a special article published in the *New England Journal of Medicine*, Mitchell Rabkin, Gerald Gillerman, and Nancy Rice described the policies developed at Beth Israel Hospital in Boston to guide "the process by which decisions not to resuscitate should be made." Although it had long been an ill-kept secret that physicians did not always attempt to resuscitate dying patients, Rabkin and his colleagues argued that there had "been little open discussion . . . of the process" by which physicians decided not to resuscitate. If Rabkin's intention was, as an accompanying editorial suggested, to take "Do Not Resuscitate" orders "out of the closet," he succeeded unambiguously.[1] Since 1976, hospital after hospital—including Outerboro and Countryside—has developed formal procedures to guide the writing of Do Not Resuscitate orders. In 1983, the President's Commission for the Study of Ethical Problems in Medicine recommended that every hospital adopt such procedures.[2] And, in 1987, New York became the first state to pass legislation enshrining a formal DNR policy in law.[3]

The purpose of these policies, at least according to the President's Commission, is straightforward: "In the absence of an established mechanism, decisionmaking might fail to meet the requirements of informed consent or the responsibility for making and carrying out the decision might be assigned to an inappropriate person."[4] Formal Do Not Resuscitate policies are in-

1. Mitchell Rabkin, Gerald Gillerman, and Nancy Rice, "Orders Not to Resuscitate," *New England Journal of Medicine* 295 (1976): 364; Charles Fried, "Terminating Life Support: Out of the Closet," *New England Journal of Medicine* 295 (1976): 390–91.

2. The President's Commission for the Study of Ethical Problems in Medicine and Biomedical and Behavioral Research (Washington: GPO, 1983), *Deciding to Forego Life-Sustaining Treatment* (Washington, DC: Government Printing Office, 1983).

3. New York State Task Force on Life and the Law, *Do Not Resuscitate Orders*, 2d ed. (New York: New York State Task Force on Life and the Law, 1988).

4. President's Commission, *Deciding to Forego Life-Sustaining Treatment*, p. 249.

tended to make what had been secret open and, in so doing, ensure the patient's (or patient's surrogate's) participation in a decision.

The widespread recourse to formal procedures represents one of the triumphs of medical ethics as a social movement. But we might be rightly skeptical of what this triumph means. Do Not Resuscitate orders have a peculiarly narrow focus, focusing as they do on efforts at cardiopulmonary resuscitation. But, as we have already seen, cardiopulmonary resuscitation is only one of many issues facing physicians and patients at the end of life. Moreover, cardiopulmonary resuscitation, in particular, is often beside the point because most patients cannot be resuscitated successfully in the event of an arrest, no matter how intense the efforts of physicians. Although there is significant variation, depending on how extensively resuscitation is attempted, most research shows that it effectively restores cardiac and respiratory function in only one out of three hospital patients and that, of those who are resuscitated, only one in three survives to discharge from the hospital, many of these with reduced abilities.[5] Thus, while I in no sense mean to denigrate those attempts at resuscitation that do succeed, it is important to recognize that most attempts do not.

Even more important, there is no evidence that the development of formal policies has in any way changed decision-making processes. As we saw in the cases of Mr. Haskell and others, the final, charted decision not to resuscitate is often almost an afterthought, duly recorded only after protracted negotiations with the family or hard-fought battles on rounds. Similarly, research at a number of New York hospitals has shown that, while the passage of New York's DNR legislation appears to have had a great deal of effect on the care with which physicians document their decisions, it has had little or no effect on the frequency with which they actually resuscitate patients.[6] It may be,

5. Susanna E. Bedell, Thomas L. Delbanco, E. Francis Cook, and Franklin H. Epstein, "Survival after Cardiopulmonary Resuscitation in the Hospital," *New England Journal of Medicine* 309 (1983): 569–76; President's Commission for the Study of Ethical Problems in Medicine and Biomedical and Behavioral Research, *Deciding to Forego Life-Sustaining Treatment,* pp. 234–35; George E. Taffet, Thomas A. Teasdale, and Robert J. Luchi, "In-Hospital Cardiopulmonary Resuscitation," *Journal of the American Medical Association* 260 (1988): 2069–72.

6. See John A. McClung and Russell S. Kamer, "Legislating Ethics: Implications of New York's Do-Not-Resuscitate Law," *New England Journal of Medicine* 323 (1990): 270–72; R. S. Kamer, E. M. Dieck, J. A. McClung, P. A. White, and S. L. Sivak, "Effects of New York State's Do-Not-Resuscitate Legislation on In-Hospital Cardiopulmonary Resuscitation Practice," *American Journal of Medicine* 88 (1990): 108–11; Judith Aronheim, "An Epidemiological Study of DNR," paper presented at the Conference on the New York State DNR Law, Union College, Sept. 11, 1990.

then, that formal DNR policies have altered only what goes in the medical chart.

But what are we to make of documentation in charts? Decisions are, in fact, made as part of a negotiated process. They are presented in medical charts, however, as something quite different. The medical chart serves two purposes. On the one hand, it is an internal hospital document, the depository of notes from the various doctors and (in a separate section) nurses who may have seen a patient. It includes a medical and social history of the patient, an account of the course of an illness, and a systematic record of vital signs and medications. In this sense, it is a tool of coordination, a convenient and reliable introduction to a case for those medical staff newly involved with a patient and a reminder even for those long involved. On the other hand, the chart is a public document, albeit in a significantly restricted sense. The chart is the property of the hospital and is, of course, confidential. Moreover, although most doctors today are willing to show charts to patients or families who ask to see them, few patients or families do.[7] The chart is, nonetheless, a public document in the sense that it is subject to review—by other physicians, by hospital administrators, and, most importantly, in litigation. And, as a public document, the chart has an audience.

Most chart notes are intended to convey information, simply and efficiently, to the rest of the medical and nursing staff. But notes about limitation of treatment are different. As one Outerboro resident explained, the Do Not Resuscitate "note itself is not written for the other house staff. I don't think the housestaff really cares what is in your note. They only care what the status of the patient is. How you word that is not really important." She suggested, moreover, that the note is written, instead, "for anyone who may review the chart," and that the "only one who would review the chart would be a lawyer or a medical review board." And another argued, about both official Do Not Resuscitate procedures in general and Do Not Resuscitate notes in particular, that, "the justification for it is legal almost exclusively, that they are worried about lawsuits being brought against the hospital." The special character of Do Not Resuscitate notes was entirely explicit in one Countryside intern's comments about a note she had written. Ann had begun her note on Mr. Novograd, a 74-year-old man with metastatic cancer, "Family (wife—Janet Novograd) & 2 daughters discussed code status requesting that

7. Richard Bernstein, Ellen M. Andrews, and Lelon Weaver, "Physician Attitudes toward Patients' Requests to Read Their Hospital Records," *Medical Care* 19 (1981): 118–21.

pt patient not be resuscitated." When I ran into her later, I asked Ann why
she had crossed out "pt" and replaced it with the word spelled out. I expected
her to find the question strange (an occupational hazard of sociology), but
she surprised me. She said she was trying to get out of the habit of using
abbreviations, particularly in DNR notes, because DNR notes are subject to
review and lots of people, even nurses, don't always know what abbreviations
stand for. Moreover, she stressed, clarity is particularly important in DNR
notes, because they are likely subjects of litigation.

There is a temptation, then, to dismiss notes about the limitation of treatment—and perhaps DNR policies more generally—as, at best, a mere formality and, at worst, obscurantist. Not only are notes written primarily for
legal documentation, but they often distort the character of decision making.
Yet to simply censure chart notes as obscurantist or to dismiss them as a
formality would be a mistake. The distinction between form and substance
is a slippery one, and forms, even obscurantist ones, often take on meanings
of their own.

Formal policies about Do Not Resuscitate orders make only limited sense
if we think of them as a means of making decisions. But they make considerably more sense if we think of them in a way that is less congenial to conventional modes of medical thought, as a type of medical ritual. From this
point of view, the significance of Do Not Resuscitate policies is not that they
shape the decisions that are made but that, in writing DNR orders, physicians are representing symbolically a set of values central to contemporary
American medicine.[8]

In the case of Kelly Connors, for example, I had asked Ken just before
one of his final conversations with Kelly's family why it mattered so much to
him that they should agree to a DNR order, especially as Ken himself
thought it highly unlikely they would be able to resuscitate her successfully.
But Ken suggested that the DNR order itself was not the point: "It tells us
something about the family. I might not bronch [bronchoscope] her." It
would, he added, be a sign of good faith on their part. The Do Not Resuscitate order—as a formal order, appropriate for a chart note—had taken on a
symbolic character.

The symbolic character of chart notes recasts their significance as legal
documents. In invoking legal considerations, I would suggest—albeit spec-
ulatively—that the Outerboro and Countryside medical staffs are not expressing a concern about potential penalties, themselves something of a chi-

8. For a discussion of rituals in medicine more generally, see Charles Bosk, "Occupational
Rituals in Patient Management," *New England Journal of Medicine* 303 (1980): 71–76.

mera, so much as they are searching for direction in an area that they find troubling and difficult. In invoking the law, the ICU physicians are invoking a system of symbols—a formal, codified representation of a normative order. This is not, of course, the language of physicians themselves. Yet, it is very much their meaning. The Do Not Resuscitate order, one Outerboro resident told me, is "a medical-legal decision [and] should be documented as such." Moreover, he added, "I don't think it's changed policy in any way." Still, while he groped for a way to express himself, he thought that formal procedures and formal notes had much of value: "It's just, it's made things a lot clearer for everyone, although initially there was a lot of resistance to it. . . . It makes life a lot easier for everyone, from attendings down to the nurses." Another resident made a similar point, stressing even more explicitly the importance of formal procedures in coping with the uncertainty endemic to medicine:

Without getting normal consent or a Do Not Resuscitate order, you would never not resuscitate a patient for fear of legal retaliation. . . . I've only lived in the era of a formal Do Not Resuscitate. I'm not sure what it was like before, but I think it's certainly clarified a patient's status most of the time. . . . When you're alone and you're a house officer, and you are dealing with a critically ill patient, you have to know whether to treat the patient aggressively or non-aggressively. You can't be vague about what needs to be done. It's just too difficult to manage a patient. So I think it's extremely important. I think it's very effective. I think it really helps you take care of the patient.

The symbolic character of Do Not Resuscitate and other orders is perhaps most apparent in their language.[9] If DNR orders were simply written pragmatically, we would expect their language to be prosaic and unadorned. But often it is not. One type of metaphor, in particular, recurs consistently. While some of the notes do state simply and explicitly that "no resuscitative efforts be made in the event of an arrest," that language is often supplanted by more metaphorical formulations. Consider, for example, the following Outerboro note:

Spoke to son about further use of extraordinary measures. Son expressed wish for father (patient) not to be subject to CPR or any further heroic measures should the need arise. Patient reportedly expressed this wish prior to his hospitalization. Son was fully aware & understood all that was explained. He was told of his father's critical condition & decision not to have him resuscitated was made. It was understood that pt. would be treated medically aggressively short of heroics—CPR, shock, etc.

The note does, to be sure, specify that the patient is not to be resuscitated.

9. Kathleen Nolan, "In Death's Shadow: The Meanings of Withholding Resuscitation," *Hastings Center Report* 17 (Oct.–Nov. 1987): 9–14.

But the note also specifies that the patient is not to be "subject" to resuscitation, a term that suggests an evaluation. Moreover, the note refers to "heroic measures" and "extraordinary measures," terms that contain an evaluation in an implicit distinction between what is routine (and therefore can be expected of physicians) and what is not routine (and, therefore, cannot be expected). These terms suggest a moral quality that goes well beyond the mere recording of an order.

Chart notes represent a recognition of the rule of law in medicine. That recognition is not explicit so much as it is implicit in the very fact that the notes are written. But other matters are explicit.

In the first instance, chart notes acknowledge the rights of patients and their surrogates. At Countryside, responsibility for decisions is usually ascribed to the family:

Discussed dismal prognosis [with] pt's daughter, who has decided [with] agreement of her sisters [on] a DNR status for their mother—no chest compressions, defibrillation, cardioversion—*They will* further *discuss* options re fluid, blood, and pressor support *and inform us* today. [Emphasis added.]

After discussing pt's condition-prognosis [with] family *they elect* for *no code* status (no CPR, defib, chemical, or vasopressors). [Emphasis added.]

At Outerboro, responsibility is also ascribed to the family, but, in response to the stricter standards of New York state law, it is more often formulated in terms of the family's representation of the wishes of the patient himself or herself:

Discussed status and prognosis with family. The wife and daughter feel that given his current poor state and prognosis, *that he would not want* and they do not want CPR performed should he suffer a cardiac arrest. All other therapy will be continued. [Emphasis added.]

After detailed discussion about pts overall medical/neurological condition, his family has agreed that the use of further "heroic" measures would be meaningless. *They feel that the pt would never have wanted to be kept alive in this manner.* We will not perform CPR or resuscitate by chemical/pharmacological means. Should the pts. condition deteriorate further, we will continue supportive measures already undertaken. [Emphasis added.]

We may, of course, be rightly skeptical that the wishes of the family are always as clear or autonomous as they seem. As we saw in chapter 11, the wishes of a family cited in notes are frequently beside the point in an actual decision-making process. Similarly, the formula, invoked frequently at Outerboro, that a surrogate is merely expressing the wishes of the patient is itself usually something of a fiction. Particularly in cases in which patients had not expressed wishes, the invocation of such wishes is often merely the language in which the family's preference is recorded. This the Outerboro housestaff openly admit. One intern remembered "distinctly" writing a Do Not Resuscitate order that said:

> "Had a long talk with so-and-so's family, someone who was *non compos mentis*, discussed all the things about it. They feel that super human or heroic treatment at this point would not, the family thinks it . . . would not be advisable, therefore." And I say, "Oh, oh" and start all over and wrote, "The family feels that *the patient* would not want heroic measures done at this point." . . . We sort of use the family in whatever role we want to, as either speaker for the patient or speaker for themselves or guardian or whatever.

The chart notes, then, at least in regard to the wishes of patients and their families, cannot be read as literal truth. They can, however, be read as symbolic truth—as the expression of an ideal.

Only an occasional note at Outerboro identifies either the patient or a member of the patient's family by name. More often, both are identified only as part of a general category. At Countryside, names are included, but only after they have been situated in a category. Thus, in the notes just cited, there are references to "wife," "daughter," and, without any specification, "family." Other notes refer simply to "husband," "son," "sister," or "brother." And, in some notes, even the patient is not mentioned by name. By assigning responsibility to a category of person rather than to a specific, named person, the notes move beyond the level of specific cases to the level of principle.

Thus, the Do Not Resuscitate orders and other chart notes express an ideal. Invocations of patients' or families' wishes are, in many cases, fictions. However, if they were merely fictions, we might expect the Outerboro and Countryside physicians to treat Do Not Resuscitate orders lightly, as little more than a nuisance. But they do not take the orders lightly, precisely because they approach the wishes of the patient with all due seriousness. Do Not Resuscitate orders evoke the value—if not the reality—of the patient's and family's rights. They should not be read as a statement of the patient's or family's wishes—although they may be such—but as an affirmation that those wishes *should* be assigned priority.

Beyond recognizing the rights of patients and the rule of law, Do Not Resuscitate orders and other chart notes are an affirmation that physicians have reached a decision and that they agree about that decision. This is not a trivial matter. For example, the following Outerboro note, referring to "agreement" among housestaff and attendings, was written after intense, week-long disagreements between housestaff and attendings over whether or not to continue giving transfusions to a 50-year-old man with an intractable gastrointestinal bleed.

In discussions [with] pt's family in light of pt's condition & poor prognosis, it was their wishes that in the light of catastrophe or CVA [cerebrovascular accident] pt should have no heroic measures taken, i.e., no CPR. *The medical housestaff & attendings remained in agreement with their decision.* [Emphasis added.]

Indeed, there is often intense disagreement, among housestaff, between housestaff and attendings, and between physicians and nurses, over how aggressively to treat patients. The simple statement in the chart that a patient is not to be resuscitated is an affirmation that, in regard to at least one type of aggressive treatment, the staff has resolved its disagreements.

At the same time, the Do Not Resuscitate order affirms the sometimes complex lines of authority within medicine. The following note, written by an Outerboro resident, refers to the agreement of consultants and Dr. Taylor, the patient's private physician. It is an acknowledgement of the right of private physicians to follow patients into the Intensive Care Unit and the priority of their responsibilities.

Have discussed pt [with] family (husband), Dr. Taylor, & consultants fully. Husband has asked that no further aggressive or invasive measures be taken & that the major focus be on the pt's comfort alone. Dr. Taylor agrees [with] above decisions by husband that no cardiopulmonary resuscitation or aggressive measures be done.

However, particularly at Outerboro, aside from references to private physicians, references to the agreement of named medical personnel (like references to named family) are notably absent. Thus, while Dr. Taylor is named, "consultants" are mentioned generically. Consider also the following note:

Discussed overall situation at length w/ patient's sister, niece (closest relatives). Family understands that patient has terminal illness and prognosis is grave. They request that CPR not be initiated for cardiac arrest & that meds to support BP (pressors) not be administered. All other supportive care to continue. *The staff of the MICU supports the decision.* Therefore, the patient is do not resuscitate. [Emphasis added.]

Here, responsibility is detached from any particular person and vested, instead, in the "staff of the MICU [Medical Intensive Care Unit]" as a corporate whole. Such a formulation insists on both the agreement of the staff and the rights of that staff, regardless of the individuals involved. In this sense, the Do Not Resuscitate order is a reaffirmation of the lines of authority in medicine—whether the authority of the private physician based on a distinctive relationship to a particular patient or the collective authority of the ICU staff based on a position in the medical division of labor.

Perhaps most important of all, the Do Not Resuscitate order represents a recognition that there are limits to what medicine is required to do. This, too, is no small matter. Medicine, as I have stressed, is caught between two sometimes conflicting values: on the one hand, an ethic of intervention and treatment; on the other hand, an injunction to do no harm. The Do Not Resuscitate order expresses, symbolically and however partially, a resolution of that conflict. It is an affirmation that there are at least some instances in which potentially therapeutic intervention may be withheld. This affirmation is made, in part, to those who might review the chart and, in part, to the patient or the patient's surrogate. But more significant, it is made among physicians themselves. It is an affirmation that active treatment is not the only value of medicine but one to be balanced against concerns of comfort and humanity.

Yet, at the same time that the formal chart note ordering treatment withheld acknowledges the limits of medicine, it defies those limits. Phillippe Aries, the French social historian, has argued in his magisterial study of Western attitudes toward death that, at least in the years since World War II, we have stripped death of its moral and spiritual significance.[10] Not for us is Little Eva ascending toward heaven, or Ivan Ilyich pondering the ultimate meaning of life in the face of death, nor even family and friends gathered around the deathbed for the moment of final benediction. For us the good death has become simply the painless death, the death that comes in sleep and allows us to say, "At least he didn't suffer." We have made death, argues Aries, a technical matter, something to be managed. We can see the effort to manage death, in part, in the work of both social scientists and physicians, like Elisabeth Kubler-Ross, who lay out predictable stages of a "dying process" and subject those stages to dispassionate analysis.[11] And we can see it even more clearly in our removal of death from the home and its relocation to the hospital or the hospice, where it can be contained, postponed, and orchestrated with all the skills of contemporary medicine. "Try to make it through the night," Ken suggested to the Countryside housestaff about a 67-year-old woman who had just been made DNR: "I wouldn't like it for the family if she expired just after I talked to them. It'd be nice psychologically, for me and for them."

10. Phillippe Aries, *The Hour of Our Death* (New York: Knopf, 1981).
11. Elisabeth Kubler-Ross, *On Death and Dying* (New York: MacMillan, 1969).

But death cannot be contained or postponed indefinitely. This the physicians at both Outerboro and Countryside are intensely aware of. "My feeling," one resident told me, "is that when they have made somebody DNR it hasn't really changed the outcome." Death is a nasty business which insists on its own way and its own timing despite the best efforts of contemporary medicine. To contemporary medicine, insistent on an ability to manage illness, it is the ultimate reproach.

The Do Not Resuscitate order is an answer to this reproach. It represents an insistence that death is not simply something that happens, but something that is allowed to happen, something about which someone has made a decision. It is in this respect that the complex provisions of DNR policies concerning who is to decide and in what circumstances make perhaps the most sense. They are an insistence that, even in the face of death, it is possible to impose order, rationality, and technique. In this sense, then, even as it represents a recognition of medicine's limits, the Do Not Resuscitate order is also an affirmation of the powers of medicine and the powers of management.

Do Not Resuscitate orders and other formal chart notes have a dual character. They are a response to and an acknowledgement of the limits of medical discretion imposed by law and the rights of patients. But, at the same time, they are a defense of medical discretion, openly acknowledging limits in public statements only to obscure the discretion exercised in what Marcia Millman has called the "backrooms of medicine." [12] They acknowledge the limits of medical technique, while at the same time they defy those limits and are themselves an instance of the triumph of technique.

Conclusion

We are accustomed to thinking of ritual as something draped in tradition, something that grows empty or hollow—that becomes mere ritual—as the values that once animated words and gestures lose touch with current realities. We are accustomed also to thinking of ritual as something that grows crescively out of a social setting, elaborated slowly and incrementally. Neither of these images holds true for the chart note documenting a decision to limit treatment. Rather, the writing of a note is something we might think of as a ritual from above. It does not simply grow out of the values of medicine. It does not simply take values already found in medical practice and then at-

12. Marcia Millman, *The Unkindest Cut* (New York: Morrow, 1977).

tempt to represent them symbolically. Instead, formal policies requiring documentation of decisions to limit treatment are an attempt to shape the values of medicine—to invite the recurrent affirmation of both the appropriateness of withholding treatment and, at the same time, of patients' rights. If such policies do not exactly change the way in which anyone makes decisions, they may do something even more significant. They may require physicians to affirm a culture in which the rights of patients are included in the values of medicine. Such policies may represent the triumph of form over substance. But substance does not always matter more than form.

13

"A Legal Thing"

Many physicians would be happy to treat the limitation of treatment as a private matter, something to be decided among themselves, their patients, and their patients' families. But limitation of treatment is not a private matter. A paradigm of how we think of life as well as how we manage death, limitation of treatment has also become very much a matter of public interest. This public interest is expressed in many ways but most importantly through law. It is through law that an otherwise diffuse public—something more than individual patients or their families—attempts to exercise some measure of control over what physicians do.

I have not, of course, been able to ignore legal questions, even in earlier chapters. In a number of instances, I have suggested that legal considerations limit the discretion of physicians. I have suggested, for example, that differences between New York and Massachusetts law help explain some of the differences between Outerboro and Countryside, particularly the tendency of physicians to limit treatment less frequently at Outerboro than at Countryside. I have suggested that legal considerations restrict the limitation of treatment to "terminally ill" patients and account for an unwillingness to withdraw some of the very same treatments that physicians otherwise withhold. And I have suggested that legal considerations permeate the kinds of notes that physicians write.

But I have also argued that legal considerations are, in effect, negotiable. The differences between Outerboro and Countryside cannot be accounted for simply by differences in state law. Physicians at both hospitals have considerable latitude in the meaning they ascribe to "terminal" and may respond to proscriptions on withdrawing some treatments by a greater caution in starting them in the first place. And the very acknowledgment of legal considerations in chart notes is, in part, a means of ignoring the law in substantive decisions.

Still, to listen to some physicians, the effects of the law on decisions to limit treatment are far more extensive than I have allowed: "I think," an Outerboro resident told me, "the vast majority of patients who are brought into ICU are brought into ICU inappropriately . . . because of the current legal situation in this country." Law does affect decisions in the ICU, particularly decisions to limit treatment. But its effects are nowhere near as extensive as such comments suggest.

To ask how the law affects decisions to limit treatment is, then, not to ask one question but to ask three. First, there is a question of what the law says. Second, there is the distinct question of how physicians respond to law in practice—in effect, how physicians negotiate attempts at regulation. Third, there is a question of why physicians believe law to be so powerful, more powerful than it is in fact.

Termination of Treatment in the Courts

In 1976 the Supreme Court of New Jersey ruled that a respirator could be removed from Karen Quinlan, a 23-year-old who, for reasons that remain unclear, had fallen into a deep and irreversible coma. Placed on a respirator in the Intensive Care Unit of Newtown Memorial Hospital, she had, according to all medical opinion, essentially no chance of emerging from what had become a persistent vegetative state. Karen's parents, articulating what they believed would have been their daughter's wishes, asked that she be removed from the respirator. Karen's physician, apparently acting under the advice of Newtown's legal counsel, refused. Karen's parents sought relief in court—and found it. When the New Jersey Supreme Court ruled in March 1976, it found "the present life-support system may be withdrawn and said action shall be without any civil or criminal liability . . . on the part of any participant."[1]

The Quinlan case, although still probably the best known, was only the first of what was to be a long list of cases bearing on termination of treatment. Thus, in the time since the Quinlan decision, case after case has specified the kinds of treatments that may be withheld or withdrawn; the conditions under which treatment may be withheld or withdrawn; who may make the decision when the patient is competent; who, when the patient is not competent; who, when the patient has never been competent; and what the role

---

1. *In re Quinlan,* 70 N.J. 10, 355 A.2d.

of the courts is to be.[2] Moreover, many of these rulings differ significantly from state to state.

The 1990 United States Supreme Court ruling in the Nancy Cruzan case did little to eliminate the confusion surrounding termination of treatment. The case—with a number of striking similarities to Quinlan—involved a then 25-year-old Missouri woman who lapsed into a persistent vegetative state after a 1983 automobile accident. As in the Quinlan case, her parents sought to terminate treatment, here consisting of artificial nutrition and hydration. The Supreme Court, however—in this unlike the New Jersey Quinlan court—ruled against the Cruzans. In so doing, the Supreme Court upheld a Missouri court's ruling, based on the state's Living Will Statute, requiring "clear and convincing evidence" of the patient's wishes. Although the Supreme Court did not reject the practice of "substituted judgment"— by which family members or other intimates make decisions on an incompetent patient's behalf—it did hold that Missouri was not constitutionally required to accept such judgment.

It might seem, then—as it does to many physicians—that termination of treatment is among the most regulated issues in medicine. It might seem, moreover, that it is the courts, above all, that have insisted on continuing treatment in circumstances in which families and physicians, left to their own devices, would sooner terminate treatment. In fact, this is far from the truth. To be sure, the courts have had a powerful effect on the practice of limiting treatment. In New York (Outerboro's home state) as well as Missouri, courts have rejected the practice of "substituted judgment." Like Missouri, New York has insisted on a strict standard of "clear and convincing evidence" that the patient, if competent, would have wanted a treatment terminated.[3] As a result, in New York, as in Missouri, it has been more difficult to limit treatment than is the case elsewhere. In most other states, however, including Massachusetts (Countryside's home state), courts have recognized substituted judgment and, as a result, have done a great deal to empower families. The Supreme Court decision in the Cruzan case leaves those decisions un-

---

2. None of this is to mention the related cases bearing on termination of treatment for newborn infants, an issue that has generated its own enormous (and often controversial) body of litigation.

3. *Matter of Storar*, 52 N.Y.2d. The criterion of "clear and convincing" evidence does, of course, leave considerable ambiguity. According to the New York State Task Force on Life and the Law (*Life-Sustaining Treatment: Making Decisions and Appointing a Health Care Agent* [New York: New York State Task Force on Life and the Law, 1987], p. 27), New York courts have, in a series of decisions since 1982, consistently "authorized the withdrawal of treatment based on testimony by family members about the patient's prior oral statements."

challenged. Most important, in New York, Massachusetts, and elsewhere, the courts have done a great deal to formalize the decision-making process surrounding the limitation of treatment. But the long legal record and the protests of some physicians notwithstanding, the courts have also allowed for considerable latitude in limiting treatment.

First, the general thrust of most court decisions has been to extend the circumstances in which treatment may be withdrawn as well as withheld. Thus, the Quinlan case made explicit that respirator care may be withdrawn. Although the Quinlan case applies only to New Jersey, other cases in virtually every state have followed the precedent set there. Both Massachusetts and New York are among the states in which court decisions have ruled that respirators may be withdrawn from respirator-dependent patients. The caution of Outerboro's legal counsel notwithstanding, the New York court of appeals declared unambiguously in the 1981 Brother Fox case that, with proper procedural safeguards, ventilator support could be discontinued.[4] Beyond allowing respirator care to be withdrawn, courts in various jurisdictions have also ruled that any number of other treatments—ranging from dialysis to feeding tubes—may be withdrawn as well as withheld.[5] In the Cruzan case, the Supreme Court implied that it, too, would not make a distinction between withdrawing and withholding treatment.

Second, when state courts have required continued treatment, they have generally done so in unusual situations, marginal to the everyday practice of medicine. For example, in the case of Storar—involving a severely retarded man with cancer—a New York court ruled that Storar's physicians must continue to provide blood transfusions, despite the mother's wish to discontinue treatments.[6] However, the critical consideration in the court's ruling was that, because of Storar's retardation, it was impossible to know what his wishes would have been. The court's decision involves an important legal principle. It distinguishes between formerly competent patients and never competent ones like Storar. But however important the principle may be to the law, its relevance to the practice of medicine in intensive care is distinctly limited. Although many, if not most, ICU patients from whom physicians want to withhold treatment are comatose and clearly no longer competent, very few (and none whatsoever in my samples at Outerboro and Countryside) have never been competent. The considerations of the Storar case, and others like it, simply do not apply to the vast majority of cases that doctors deal with

4. *Matter of Storar.*
5. See, above all, *Matter of Conroy,* 98 N.J. 321, 486 A.2d.
6. *Matter of Storar.*

every day. "Most of the cases," John, the director of the Outerboro unit, observed of recent legal decisions, "have very little effect."

Third, most court cases have been marginal to the everyday practice of intensive care medicine in still another sense. As I pointed out earlier, the most frequent type of decision to limit treatment is the Do Not Resuscitate order. But there have been precious few court cases involving DNR orders in particular.[7] Moreover, when courts have addressed DNR orders, they have generally treated them more permissively than other types of treatment limitation, subsuming them directly under the common law doctrine of informed consent. Although I do not mean to understate the ambiguity surrounding the legal status of DNR orders, even in New York substituted judgments seemed to enjoy a quasi-legal status denied them in other circumstances.[8] (The ambiguity surrounding DNR orders in New York state disappeared with the passage, in 1987, of legislation explicitly legalizing substituted judgments in such orders. The legislation has been in effect only since April of 1988, after the completion of my research at Outerboro.)

Fourth, the courts have generally (and self-consciously) attempted to restrict their own role. Thus, the courts have ruled consistently that they are not the appropriate forum for making decisions about termination of treatment. One apparent exception is the Saikewicz case, a case, like Storar, involving a severely retarded adult man. In that case, a Massachusetts court seemed to imply that all termination of treatment cases required judicial approval. But after a brief experiment in which judges found themselves interrupted and awakened by frequent and insistent demands to rule on one case or another, a second Massachusetts court quickly overruled the lower court. Thus, most termination of treatment cases—in Massachusetts and elsewhere—do not have to be adjudicated.

I do not mean to suggest, however, that the effects of law on the limitation of treatment are entirely a matter of physicians' (or hospital administrators') imagination. While courts have generally taken a permissive stance in regard to substantive issues in limitation of treatment, they have taken a far more restrictive stance in regard to procedures. Most important, courts have generally acted to empower patients or (even in New York, at least in regard to DNR orders) patients' families. Thus, while the courts have permitted treat-

7. One of the exceptions is a Massachusetts case, *In re Dinnerstein*, 380 N.E.2d 134, which explicitly accepted both the practice of writing DNR orders and the use of substituted judgment in the case of incompetent patients.

8. New York State Task Force on Life and the Law, *Do Not Resuscitate Orders* (New York: New York State Task Force on Life and the Law, 1986).

ment to be limited in an increasing number of circumstances, they have not mandated that treatment must be limited. That decision, in the court's view, is to be left to the patient or someone acting on the patient's behalf. In the Quinlan case, for example, the court did not order Karen Quinlan's respirator removed. Rather, the court limited itself to a procedural order, ruling that Joseph Quinlan had the right to select a physician who would comply with what he believed would have been his daughter's wishes. Thus, in sharp contrast to their generally permissive stance in extending the types of treatments that may be withheld or withdrawn (and to their self-restraint about their own role in decisions), courts have insisted on the priority of the patient's own wishes. In this sense, the courts have shifted the balance of influence not from the physician to themselves, but from the physician to either the patient or those best able to speak for the patient—most often the patient's family.

Principles and Practice

The law is one thing. Its effect on the behavior of physicians is quite another. This distinction is a version of what Max Weber had in mind when he demarcated, in characteristically turgid prose, the legal from the sociological concept of the law. A legal or juristic conception of the law addresses "the correct meaning of propositions the content of which constitutes an order supposedly determinative for the conduct of a defined group of persons." In contrast, a sociological conception addresses "what *actually* happens in a group owing to the *probability* that persons . . . subjectively consider certain norms as valid."[9] The distinction is an important one. A juristic concept addresses what the law says. A sociological concept addresses the effects of the law on human action. While there have been a great many commentaries on what the law says about limiting treatment (the juristic approach), there have been very few that attempt to make sense of the actual effect of those laws on physicians.

Consider, for example, Mr. Jameson. The remarkable discussion that accompanied his case justifies an extended account.

Lewis Jameson had been in Outerboro for nearly a month when he suffered a respiratory arrest in the Intensive Care Unit. Ninety-one years old, with a history of both severe heart disease and prostate cancer, now unres-

9. Max Weber, *Economy and Society* (Berkeley: University of California Press, 1968), vol. 1, p. 311.

ponsive and in renal failure, Jameson seemed to the ICU staff exactly the sort of patient whose treatment should be limited. To be sure, Mark, one of the attendings on the case, acknowledged that they could not be "absolutely certain" Jameson would not recover. Yet, faced with Jameson's renal failure, none of the ICU staff were enthusiastic about dialysis. Mark asked if Jameson had any family. Told that he had a sister, he suggested: "We should hang the crepe. Make her understand that we aren't optimistic." But Jameson's sister, a former rehabilitation therapist ("She's smart; you can't trick her"), could not be convinced. Despite the urging of her brother's physicians, she insisted that Jameson receive dialysis for his renal failure as well as vasopressors to manage his blood pressure. Now the ICU staff disagreed among themselves—not about whether dialyzing Jameson made good sense medically (all agreed that it did not) but about whether they should honor the sister's wishes. Mark argued that they should not: "The man is terminal, and medical maneuvers won't have any effect." But Lynn, a resident, was uncomfortable with Mark's position: "If you think we have the right not to do what she wants, show me where that's written." Now Mark was uncomfortable: "She just doesn't want to make the decision." And the other attending added, "I still don't think he needs pressors." But Lynn continued: "We agree. It's a matter of what hospital policy is. . . . It's a legal thing. She's made very clear what she wants. She understands that there's no chance in the long run." Mark countered that, if Mr. Jameson's sister asked the ICU staff to use a particular drug, they would not honor her request—that that would be a matter of what is "medically indicated." Lynn was not satisfied. The sister, she argued, understood Mr. Jameson's condition: "She wants to prolong this state. We're saying it's not worth preserving." And that, she continued, is not "a medical issue." "I wish," she concluded, "the family didn't have the final say. But in 1987 they do. . . . There are two moral issues. One is if it's right to do. The other is if it's right when the family wants it." Now neither attending was satisfied. The one who had been quiet throughout most of the discussion said, "I still think you're concerned with what we're allowed to do," but added that he thought the district attorney would not take an interest, if that were her concern. But Mark's position was different: "It's a political decision. There are some people who . . . think the state should make personal decisions, and there are other people who think society delegates that responsibility." Mr. Jameson continued to receive dialysis until he was transferred to the respirator room.

The Jameson case neatly ties together a number of themes. For reasons I discussed earlier, the ICU staff is unhappy at having to treat a patient they believe to be terminal. They acknowledge uncertainty. They negotiate with the family. But the case also adds something distinctive—an explicit discussion of the patient's family, framed around that family's legal empowerment. The law is not mentioned to invoke the possibility of coercion. There is an explicit recognition that criminal charges are unlikely, and the possibility of malpractice is not mentioned. Neither is there anything approaching a detailed discussion of a legal case. Allusions to the law are vague and general. Instead, the "legal thing" is invoked as a general framework which vests the right to decide in the hands of the patient's family—and even though the rights of the family to decide for the patient were highly ambiguous in New York at the time of the discussion. There is no disagreement between Mark and Lynn about what the law requires. Rather, they disagree about whether there is a moral obligation for physicians to honor what they see as the law's empowerment of the family.

Mark (and some of the other attendings and residents) is prepared to deny a legal obligation to respect Mrs. Jameson's wishes, arguing either that "society" has delegated the responsibility for medical decisions to physicians or that physicians should practice medicine without regard to legal considerations. It is a position that verges on principled civil disobedience. Others, however, are not so bold. Even if they are prepared to contest particular choices made by or for particular patients and to argue that some decisions are properly medical, they are not prepared to challenge what they understand to be the legal rights of patients and families. ("I wish the family didn't have the final say. But in 1987 they do.") What is at stake is the legitimacy of legal authority—and, by implication, the legitimacy of medical authority.

Physicians and the Law

Although the law has altered the procedures by which treatment may be limited, it has taken a generally permissive stance toward the substantive issues surrounding that practice. Physicians, however, often chafe at what seems to them an overbearing legal system—resenting both (real) procedural restrictions and (largely imaginary) substantive restrictions. Particularly at Outerboro, where cautious legal counsel (although not the law itself) has resulted in a prohibition on withdrawing respirator care, physicians are often deeply resentful of legal regulation.

To be sure, some Outerboro physicians would like to claim that the law has no effect on their behavior, that they practice medicine without regard to legal considerations. Dennis, the Outerboro unit director, in particular, frequently insisted on this point during rounds: Discussing a patient who, according to an intern's report, may have left a living will, he said, "Who cares legal? If we really believe the patient meant what he said, we can honor his wishes." Responding to a resident's suggestion that the law did not permit withdrawing ventilator support, he said, "You should just leave the law out of this. It's hard enough to practice medicine without practicing law, too." And in a similar situation, he said, "Our goal here is not to practice law. It's hard enough to practice medicine." Or, as a resident put it when I asked her if legal considerations ever influenced her decisions, "I am not a lawyer."

The very vehemence, however, with which some of the Outerboro doctors deny the influence of the law may be an instance of their protesting too much. Consider the resident who asserted that she was "not a lawyer." As I pressed her, she qualified her claim. Legal considerations, she still insisted, did not make a difference in "the way I act." But she quickly added, "I think it makes a difference in the way the rest of the people around here act." And she continued:

I think that there are certainly times. . . . I most vividly remember being told by the chairman of the department that we had to accept the patient transferred from the neurologic [service] who was clearly essentially dead. And it was clearly for medical documentation, for legal documentation, that everything had been done. . . . That was purely legal documentation, and that I object to strongly. . . . I think that there is almost a clash sometimes between what I would do medically and what I am told I am supposed to do legally.

What seems likely is that claims to the effect that law has no influence should be read normatively rather than factually—as claims that the law should not have an influence rather than as claims that it does not.

Other Outerboro residents and attendings are more explicit. Indeed, for many, a concern about legal considerations is the fundamental explanation for aggressive treatment and for "torture." Two residents:

If I were to pick up on something that I would do differently, I think . . . people are too aggressive a lot of times, and I think that part of that is legal. . . . A lot of it, it's not mentioned. I guess I would probably be inclined not to be quite as aggressive as we are because of that. . . . Some of the medical tests that are done are probably a little over zealous.

The situations you're describing, where we're piece by piece stopping doing things, should be the easy ones because those are the situations where the patient is basically dead and the family wants nothing done. We want nothing done, and we're kind of trying to deal with what we see as the law. . . . So kind of bit by bit so it won't look so bad, it won't look like we're just turning things off, we are turning things off. I think that's a problem with the way the legal system is right now, that we have to do it that way. Generally, there the problem is just legal.

Thus, legal regulation appears to the Outerboro physicians as both powerful and unwelcome.

At Countryside the situation is somewhat different. John, the unit director there, openly acknowledges the limits of the law on physicians' discretion but resists exaggeration. "You are influenced by the court cases and the rulings, but you still have to be a functioning physician." Rather than ascribing pervasive influence to the law, John understands its requirements as limited primarily to a few specific mandates. On a number of occasions he has even actively sought legal intervention, turning to the court to seek legal guardianship prior to limiting the treatment of incompetent or no longer competent patients without families available to act as surrogate decision makers. Ken, too, easily acknowledged the law's influence in specific situations. He recalled that in one case he was ordering an electroencephalogram of a brain-dead patient not for diagnostic but for legal reasons. In the case of an unresponsive patient without a family he argued that a respirator could not be withdrawn without a definitive diagnosis because of "the law of the land." He suggested in a third case that hydration of a dying patient not be begun, because Massachusetts law does not allow its discontinuation, once begun.

Yet, even at Countryside, although the limits of the law are openly acknowledged, they are far from welcome. John, for example, complained on a number of occasions that the legal climate in Massachusetts is particularly "antidoctor." And Ken—in this, unlike John—insisted that, in cases of incurable, incompetent patients without surrogates, "I never seek legal guardianship," preferring to make unilateral decisions without court intervention. Moreover, many of the Countryside housestaff expressed a hostility to the law virtually indistinguishable from that of their counterparts at Outerboro: "The whole problem with medicine today," one intern told me, "is that it's too litigious."

Nowhere is the physician's resentment of legal regulation more evident than in regard to malpractice. This resentment is expressed, in part, in an occasional invocation of malpractice as an explanation for aggressive treatment. An Outerboro resident: "I think, unfortunately, because of a fear of being sued at a later date, most physicians really are willing to provide every available technology to a patient to the point of death, when there isn't any question or doubt of a patient's getting better." More often, though, resentment toward malpractice is expressed in the form of pointed jokes. One day, for example, one of the Outerboro residents interrupted rounds to say that the nurses were "going crazy" about Mr. Stone, an AIDS patient, because he was arresting and there was not a formal order to withhold resuscitation. An attending said he would write the order. As he handed the chart back to the resident, he joked, "I'll give them my lawyer's number, too." One of the residents began to sing the jingle from advertisements for Jacobi & Myers (a law firm that advertises widely on television, offering to handle malpractice cases), and an intern laughingly added that he had two patients in the Cardiac Care Unit named Jacobi and Myers. All this was done in good humor. But, as is often the case in jokes, there was, at the same time, an unmistakably critical tone in the laughter.

At both Outerboro and Countryside, then, albeit with different emphases, the law seems both unwelcome and powerful. Its power does not, however, emanate from a fear of its penalties. To be sure, Ken in one instance, criticized an intern's equivocation: "If you present a patient like this and think he's brain dead, you can't say 'not really' to a judge. You'll go to jail." Similarly, an Outerboro resident, in explaining why he did not withdraw treatments, claimed simply, "I don't want to go to jail." Such concerns have no doubt been exacerbated by the threats of some local prosecutors to pursue cases in which treatment has been withheld and, especially in New York, by a 1982 grand jury investigation of Do Not Resuscitate orders in a Queens hospital. But these considerations notwithstanding, the concerns are very much exaggerated. In very few cases have criminal charges even been brought against health professionals for withholding treatment. The Queens grand jury, for example, did not find grounds for pursuing the 1982 case.[10] And, equally important, there have been "no successful criminal prosecutions for the withdrawal of life-sustaining treatment."[11]

Neither is malpractice, a matter of civil rather than criminal law, a significant threat in fact rather than imagination. Malpractice suits for limiting treatment are nearly as rare as criminal cases. There may be malpractice suits over the events leading up to the limitation of treatment. But because malpractice is based on damages and because damages are likely to be slight for a patient already incurable, the limitation of treatment is a distinctly unpromising site for such litigation. As one attending explained, "Lawsuits are expensive—$100,000—which you won't get for a terminal patient with AIDS."

10. New York State Task Force on Life and the Law, *Life-Sustaining Treatment*, p. 10.
11. Hastings Center, *Guidelines on the Termination of Life-Sustaining Treatment and the Care of the Dying* (Bloomington: Indiana University Press, 1987), p. 4.

None of the attendings or housestaff at Countryside had been to court for cases concerning limitation of treatment except for those instances of seeking legal guardianship mentioned earlier. At Outerboro, to the best of my knowledge, none of the attendings or housestaff had ever been to court over any such case.

Criminal prosecution is virtually unheard of around limitation of treatment. Malpractice is at most a distant possibility. The law does not coerce physicians with threats of penalties—with threats of jail or financial loss. Yet legal considerations continue to disquiet the physicians at both Outerboro and Countryside. As one Outerboro attending explained, in the absence of legal considerations "I might not change any of the decisions I make, but I would probably be more comfortable doing it." Some part of the physicians' disquiet stems from the uncertainty that the law creates. As one Outerboro resident explained, in an insightful comment, "The law doesn't allow us to remove therapies. Or at least we're not sure enough that we can remove therapies that we feel comfortable doing it." In short, the law adds legal uncertainty to medical uncertainty and what I have called social uncertainty. Yet even legal uncertainty does not explain the intensity of physicians' responses to the law. What is at stake, I would suggest, is not coercion but a symbolic representation of the limits of medicine's authority.

It is entirely to the point, in this respect, that physicians' knowledge of the law is typically vague and allusive. At Countryside, John—but only John—did occasionally mention specific court cases. Yet even he brought to the examination of legal issues little of the meticulous care that he brought to medical questions. As he readily acknowledged, he rarely consults with the hospital attorney: "When you hear these cases discussed . . . I'm not going to do anything pro-active. I'll wait. I certainly could call the hospital lawyer, but the hospital lawyer is going to give us the same advice." Even after the Saikewicz case, which briefly required Massachusetts physicians to consult frequently with courts, he made little effort to seek direct legal counsel about his obligations: "We talked about it," he explained, "in the lunchroom."

At Outerboro, at no point in the entire course of my research did I hear a doctor discuss any specific legal case, save for one passing mention of a malpractice suit that had resulted in a multi-million-dollar settlement—a matter of some interest but with no particular relevance to any of the issues that animate intensive care. The absence of such discussion is all the more striking in that a New York appellate court, in the *Matter of Delio,* issued the first decision in the state allowing the discontinuation of artificial nutrition and hydration during the course of my research at Outerboro.[12] Yet I did not hear a single physician so much as mention the case.

For their own purposes, the physicians at Countryside and Outerboro do not need—and certainly do not seek—a detailed knowledge of the law. Rather, they assimilate the law into a cultural framework, both a source of and roughly parallel to what I earlier called a culture of rights. If the culture of rights contains an acknowledgment of the empowerment of patients to set the broad direction of their care, it derives in part from an acknowledgment of the ability of courts and legislatures to erect a framework within which physicians and patients alike make decisions. And just as the culture of rights is compatible with resistance to patients' decisions in specific circumstances, so, too, it is compatible with resistance to legal obligations in specific circumstances. Where physicians' response to law, in particular, differs from their response to the culture of rights more generally, however, is in the degree of legitimacy they grant to their claims. In general (and no matter how bitter their resistance in specific circumstances), physicians accept the empowerment of patients as right and proper. In contrast, physicians respond with resentment to the intrusions of courts and legislatures. This response to the law should not be understood as a matter of practice so much as one of ideology. Physicians are not concerned about specific and limited legal obligations. Instead, they are concerned with the bases of medical discretion. From this perspective, the point is not what the law says but the simple fact that it says anything at all. Even if the courts eventually permit physicians a wide range of discretion, this discretion now depends, implicitly, on the indulgence of the courts. Physicians are angry about—and often overestimate—the effects of the law on the limitation of treatment. But they are not angry so much because the law limits their discretion as because the very presence of the law implies that that discretion is not theirs by right.

Conclusion

The law does alter the procedures by which physicians decide to terminate treatment. In particular, courts have attempted to increase the influence of patients, or, in some cases, their families, on those decisions. Law has not, however, restricted the situations in which physicians may limit treatment, except at the margins of medical practice. Moreover, even in its effort to empower patients and families, the law has not entirely succeeded. To be

12. New York State Task Force on Life and the Law, *Life-Sustaining Treatment*, p. 27.

sure, some physicians honor the law's mandate, in spirit as well as letter. Others do not. Nonetheless, physicians often resent the law deeply and ascribe to it an influence unwarranted by court findings. In this, physicians are fighting a battle of symbols. They are bracing to defend their jurisdiction—the legitimacy of medical authority—not so much in substance as against a counterclaim that is, at the moment, more potential than real. Because physicians resent any interference with their discretion, they exaggerate the limited interference that the law does represent. The irony is that physicians, in their resentment of legal interference, make the law's influence greater than it would otherwise be.

14

The Last Bed

Triage is different. Consider again the cases of Kelly Connors and Scranton Haskell.

Kelly Connors had been in Countryside's Intensive Care Unit for nearly two months. For the first of those months she had been a favorite of the doctors and nurses, in large part because her acute kidney disease seemed reversible. But at the end of her first month in the unit, Kelly had arrested and not wakened up again. With each day she remained unresponsive, the doctors caring for her grew more pessimistic and more insistent that she should be made DNR. But her mother and father and fiancé resisted. Finally, after several weeks of frustration, Ken, the attending who had been the physician of record for the full length of Kelly's stay and who had grown close to Kelly's family, threatened to withdraw from the case. After a long talk with the family, he returned to the unit just before teaching rounds. He explained that he had told Kelly's family that she was taking up a bed someone else could use better. Norm, the teaching attending, was skeptical that such an argument would do much to convince a family as relentlessly optimistic as the Connorses. But when Ken raised the possibility of sending Kelly to the floor, on a respirator, as a full code, Norm agreed: "The family doesn't have any say in that."

Scranton Haskell was a classic "train wreck." He had entered the Outerboro ICU three weeks earlier with severe heart disease, a gastrointestinal bleed, and an underlying cancer that was diagnosed a few days after his admission. After two weeks Haskell lapsed into an unresponsive state, the result of either a stroke or the spread of cancer to his brain. The ICU physicians thought there was nothing more to be done, but Haskell's wife did not agree, insisting that her husband receive dialysis and remain a "full code." Still, when Dennis, one of the attendings, wondered out loud if Haskell were a candidate for the respirator room, the four-bed step-down unit, the other attending agreed immediately with no thought at all of Mrs. Haskell's wishes. But the respirator room was full and the idea was tabled. Three days later, one of the residents succeeded in extubating Haskell. Dennis greeted the accomplishment with enthusiasm: "So he doesn't even have to go to a respirator room. You're a genius." Mr. Haskell was sent to the floor later that afternoon. His wife was informed of the transfer, but she was not consulted about it.

Triage—the assignment of priorities for admission to or transfer from intensive care—is entirely explicit at Outerboro and Countryside. The practice may not be widely discussed with patients or their families, but neither is it hidden. Indeed, at Outerboro a pamphlet prepared by the nursing staff for visitors to the unit states unambiguously that patients may be "transferred from the MICU to a regular patient floor . . . if the bed in the MICU is needed for a more acutely ill patient." At Countryside, unit policy is equally clear: "All patients may be triaged as required by staff members of the Critical Care Medicine Service according to established policy." Moreover, at both hospitals occasional physicians, by and large the more conscientious among them, may explain to concerned family that a husband or mother or child has been transferred from the unit because someone else needs a bed there more. Physicians make no secret of triage—to families, patients, or anyone else. But this is by way of courtesy and honesty. It is not to invite participation.

Decisions to withhold or withdraw treatment, to write a Do Not Resuscitate order, even to send a patient for a test, are all—as I have shown over the last several chapters—often matters of long and complex negotiations among doctors, patients, nurses, and families. But triage involves a decision—or, more accurately, a set of decisions—that doctors reserve to themselves.

In the decisions to transfer Connors and Haskell, there is no hint of the equivocations and tensions that characterized the decisions whether to make them DNR, whether to treat aggressively. There is no deference, real or feigned, to the wishes of Haskell's wife or Connors's father. Here, instead, is the bold assertion of the physicians' right to decide, on their own and without consultation, who will stay in the unit and who will leave.

The reasons for the difference between triage and other decisions are easy enough to understand. Decisions about withholding and withdrawing, about DNR orders and tests, are all formulated exclusively in terms of the best interests of a single patient. In contrast, triage entails weighing the claims of one patient against those of another. Where it is hard, both morally and ideologically, to deny (at least completely) the right of a patient or a patient's family to speak in his or her own best interest, it is relatively easy to deny a patient the right to judge his or her own needs against those of other patients. In decisions to limit treatment, the physician can do no more than claim to understand the patient's interests better than does the patient himself or herself. In contrast, in triage the physician can occupy the moral high ground as the disinterested defender of the common interest against the demands of very much self-interested patients and families.

Not only are patients and their families absent from the clinical debates surrounding triage, but, perhaps more surprisingly, so, too, has the law been absent from the public policy debates. In stark contrast to the seemingly endless cases addressing one or another aspect of limiting treatment, one case alone has addressed directly the matter of triage. Moreover, in equally stark contrast to the persistent emphasis on patient autonomy in cases bearing on withholding and withdrawing treatment, the 1972 Von Stetina case implicitly assigned determinations of who would most benefit from intensive care to the medical judgment of physicians.[1]

Neither have ethicists attempted with any great zeal to interfere with the discretion of physicians in these matters. In part, this is due to ethicists' general lack of attention, until quite recently, to questions of triage. There was a flurry of interest in triage among ethicists in the mid–1960s, primarily in response to the limited availability of kidney dialysis. But that interest waned with the passage in 1972 of a special amendment to the Social Security Act that made dialysis virtually universally available.[2] Only in the past several years have ethicists, undoubtedly in response to growing concerns with the costs of medicine and a new sense of the finite character of medical resources, assigned triage (and the allocation of resources more generally) a prominent place on their intellectual agenda.[3] Yet, even in these circumstances, they have suggested little that would threaten the preeminence of physicians in clinical decisions.

While I do not wish to overemphasize the degree of consensus among ethicists (always risky), it nonetheless seems clear that they have, for the most part, rejected two principles of triage that would present such a threat. First, an insistence on "social worth" as a criterion for triage would place decisions in the hands of lay people best able to evaluate the contribution of a patient to the community. But ethicists have rejected social worth—a criterion that might give a wife and mother of five preference over an unmarried, childless woman or a policeman preference over a criminal—as both impracticable

1. Barbara R. Grumet, "Legal Perspectives on the Allocation of Intensive Care Resources," in Martin A. Strosberg, I. Alan Fein, and James D. Carroll, eds., *Rationing of Medical Care for the Critically Ill*, pp. 76–79 (Washington, DC: Brookings Institution, 1989).

2. On dialysis and the ethical issues surrounding it, see Renee Fox and Judith Swazey, *The Courage to Fail*, 2d ed. (Chicago: University of Chicago Press, 1978).

3. See, for example, Henry J. Aaron and William B. Schwartz, *The Painful Prescription* (Washington, DC: Brookings Institution, 1984); H. Tristram Englehardt, "Allocating Scarce Medical Resources and the Availability of Organ Transplantation," *New England Journal of Medicine* 311 (1984): 66–71; H. Tristram Englehardt and Michael Rie, "Intensive Care Units, Scarce Resources, and Conflicting Principles of Justice," *Journal of the American Medical Association* 255 (1986): 1159–64.

and deeply offensive to democratic values. Second, an insistence on random selection or a policy of "first come, first served" would establish mechanical principles that would place decisions in the hands of administrators. But ethicists have also rejected random selection, seeing it as a flight from responsibility. Rather, ethicists—albeit with many variants and with all due qualifications—have tended to argue that triage, at least on a clinical level, should be based primarily on medical utility, just as it is in battlefield settings. Battlefield triage—the proximate source of the term as it is applied in contemporary medicine, of the sort made famous in "MASH,"[4] and a standard operating procedure in the United States military since at least World War I[5]—implies a clear mandate. Separate, on the one hand, those without immediate needs for medical attention and, on the other hand, those beyond the help of medicine from those most likely to benefit. So, too, could ICU triage select those most likely to benefit from a unit's special services. Exclude those who will do well without the ICU. Exclude those who will do poorly even with the ICU. And give priority for admission and retention to those patients for whom the respirator care and intensive nursing that are the hallmarks of ICUs might make a life-saving difference.[6] Most ethicists find this a sound principle. It is also a principle which places the critical decisions in the hands of physicians, uniquely expert in precisely the prognostic skills essential to the determination of medical utility.

Law and ethics have joined to turn triage back to the physicians. And to the physicians—at least those who have taken part in public discussions of the issue—triage becomes a technical question. Grant that triage decisions should be made on the basis of medical utility. Then the problem becomes the development of reliable prognostics. More specifically, at least according to some researchers, the problem becomes one of developing systematic predictive models. In the words of William Knaus, director of the Intensive Care

4. The term comes originally from a French word for procedures used in sorting coffee beans. It was later applied to battlefield situations by the great rationalizers of Napoleonic France and adopted as official procedure in the United States army during World War I. It is, of course, quite likely that the principles underlying triage were applied in France, the United States, and elsewhere well before the term came into use and well before the practice had been systematized.

5. James F. Childress, "Triage in Neonatal Intensive Care: The Limitations of a Metaphor," *Virginia Law Review* 69 (1983): 547–63. On the distinction between military and civilian triage, see Daniel Teres, "Triage: An Everyday Occurrence in the Intensive Care Unit," in Strosberg et al., eds., *Rationing*, pp. 70–75.

6. Albert G. Mulley, "The Allocation of Resources for Medical Intensive Care," in President's Commission for the Study of Ethical Problems in Medicine and Biomedical and Behavioral Research, *Securing Access to Health Care*, vol. 3: *Appendices, Empirical, Legal, and Conceptual Studies* (Washington, DC: Government Printing Office, 1983), pp. 285–312.

Unit Research Program at George Washington University and one of the leading scholars in the effort to rationalize triage decisions, triage that is "democratic and scientifically rigorous" requires nothing less than "probability estimates that are based on objective, accurate, and reproducible estimates of risk, need, and potential benefit for intensive care."[7] The estimates that Knaus and others have developed are indeed sophisticated, with complex provisions for length of stay, prior medical condition, and acuity of condition at the time of admission. The predictive models are technically and scientifically imposing. They are also sociologically naive.

It is all very well and good to develop "precise criteria governing admission and discharge from intensive care units."[8] But such criteria matter not at all if they are ignored, for what is left out of the predictive models—as well

7. William A. Knaus, "Criteria for Admission to the Intensive Care Unit," in Strosberg et al, eds., *Rationing*, p. 47. See also George E. Thibault, Albert G. Mulley, G. Otto Barnett, Richard L. Goldstein, Victoria A. Reder, Ellen L. Sherman, and Erik R. Skinner, "Medical Intensive Care: Indications, Interventions, and Outcomes," *New England Journal of Medicine* 302 (1980): 938–42; Edward W. Campion, Albert G. Mulley, Richard L. Goldstein, G. Otto Barnett, and George E. Thibault, "Medical Intensive Care for the Elderly: A Study of Current Use, Costs, and Outcomes," *Journal of the American Medical Association* 246 (1981): 2052–56; William Knaus, Douglas Wagner, Elizabeth Draper, Diane Lawrence, and Jack Zimmerman, "The Range of Intensive Care Services Today," *Journal of the American Medical Association* 246 (1981): 2711–16; William Knaus, Elizabeth Draper, and Douglas Wagner, "The Use of Intensive Care: New Research Initiatives and Their Implications for National Health Policy," *Milbank Memorial Fund Quarterly* 61 (1983): 561–83; William A. Knaus, Jack E. Zimmerman, Douglas P. Wagner, Elizabeth A. Draper, and Diane E. Lawrence, "APACHE—Acute Physiology and Chronic Health Evaluation: A Physiologically Based Classification System," *Critical Care Medicine* 9 (1981): 591–97; William A. Knaus, Elizabeth A. Draper, Douglas P. Wagner, and Jack E. Zimmerman, "An Evaluation of Outcome from Intensive Care in Major Medical Centers," *Annals of Internal Medicine* 104 (1986): 410–18; William Knaus, Douglas Wagner, and Elizabeth Draper, "Development of APACHE," *Critical Care Medicine* 17 (1989): S181–S185; Daniel Teres, Stanley Lemeshow, Jill Spitz Avrunin, and Harris Pastides, "Validation of the Mortality Prediction Model for ICU Patients," *Critical Care Medicine* 15 (1987): 208–12; John Rapoport, Daniel Teres, Stanley Lemeshow, and Donald Harris, "Timing of Intensive Care Unit Admission in Relation to ICU Outcome," *Critical Care Medicine* 18 (1990): 1231–35. Most of the proponents of predictive models have expressed considerable caution about their use in decisions about the admission and discharge of individual patients. However, there are clear indications that, whatever the intent behind the models, "the resulting predicted probabilities of outcome will eventually be used by physicians as part of their information base for treatment decisions for individual patients." William Knaus and Douglas Wagner, "Individual Patient Decisions," *Critical Care Medicine* 17 (1989): S204.

8. Knaus, "Criteria," p. 45. For one effort to measure the effect of these criteria on admissions, see Kim A. Eagle, Albert G. Mulley, Steven J. Skates, Victoria A. Reder, Britain W. Nicholson, Jayne O. Sexton, G. Octo Barnett, and George E. Thibault, "Length of Stay in the Intensive Care Unit: Effects of Practice Guidelines and Feedback," *Journal of the American Medical Association* 264 (1990): 992–96.

as of the ethical reflections on triage—is any sense of the socially structured pressures operating on physicians, individually and collectively, to admit or discharge one patient or another. What is left out is any sense of the social structures that generate advocacy and disinterest, that generate indifference to some patients and commitments to others strong enough to overwhelm any objective reading of probability estimates. It is a central contention of this chapter that the influence of such structures on actual triage decisions systematically undermines the promise of unbiased "science" implicit in predictive models.

Underlying predictive models is what might be called a utilitarian ethic—in which the needs of different patients are weighed against each other in the name of the greatest good for the greatest number. But in their rush to develop more sophisticated models to guide triage decisions, many of the physicians engaged in that enterprise seem to have forgotten just how novel such a utilitarian ethic is in medicine. Still, it is novel, as is its expression in triage. At the core of triage is an acknowledgment—in behavior, if not always in words—that the physician's responsibility to an individual may be tempered by concerns outside the purely dyadic relationship of doctor and patient.

While the Outerboro and Countryside physicians have few doubts that triage decisions should be their own, they are not entirely convinced (especially at Outerboro) that they should be making such decisions at all. Consider the following exchange about Scranton Haskell, whose case I discussed at length in chapter 11 and again at the beginning of this chapter, just two days before he was transferred from the unit.

Mark was frustrated. "Someday we're going to have an accountant in here and we're going to have to justify what we're doing." But Dennis answered quickly and sharply, "Not while I'm here." Mark explained, "I'm not talking about a financial accountant. I mean an effort accountant. We have a twelve-bed unit." But even this was not enough to satisfy Dennis: "While we're talking about *him*, we're talking about *him*."

The point of contention between Mark and Dennis was not about who should make a triage decision. Neither was it a question of whether Haskell belonged in the unit. Dennis was, in fact, as anxious to see him transferred out as was Mark, and both were, at that point, simply waiting for a bed in the respirator room to become available. Rather, the point of contention was whether considerations of triage should be entertained at all. Mark was prepared to transfer Haskell because of the disproportionate share of ICU resources he was consuming. He was prepared to transfer him in favor of other, potential patients who might benefit more from unit care. Dennis was also prepared to transfer Haskell, but only on grounds of the best interests of the patient himself. He was unwilling to allow considerations about other patients to interfere with his advocacy for Haskell.

The same disagreement was echoed in interviews, at least at Outerboro. One resident told me, "The patients who are in the unit are patients who are there and who you obviously do have responsibility for. To assume that you have responsibility for someone who may not exist is obviously ridiculous." But another thought differently. "I think that we have a responsibility to all patients. . . . We shouldn't adopt people as our pets. Because they're here, they were here first, they get to stay here forever? No. I think that ICUs are a community resource."

What is at stake, then, in the practice of triage is nothing less than a very general conception of the doctor-patient relationship. American medicine, almost uniquely, has been organized to maximize "Hippocratic individualism"—the role of the physician as an advocate for the individual patient. As the economist Jeffrey Harris has argued, a patient's "purchase" of a doctor's services does not involve the purchase of a specific procedure but a "general guarantee to be given appropriate medical care." As a result, Harris argues, the "doctor-patient relation creates a much stronger expectation of fidelity than is present in other agent-client arrangements." Moreover, as "an implicit part of his contract," the physician "is supposed to take a single-minded devotion to his assignment."[9] In contrast, triage implicates the physician in a role as a gatekeeper, weighing the needs of potential patients against a "single-minded devotion" to those actual patients currently in his or her care. Triage, then, requires the substitution of a utilitarian ethic for Hippocratic individualism. In this sense, what is more significant than the ways in which triage decisions are made is the mere fact that they are made at all.

There have, to be sure, long been pockets of medical practice in which single-minded devotion to the individual patient has, at least, been questioned. In military medicine, public health, and medical research—albeit in each case for different reasons—commitments to an organization or to health in general have long competed with commitment to the welfare of the individual patient.[10] The practice of triage in intensive care, however, brings

9. Jeffrey Harris, "The Internal Organization of Hospitals: Some Economic Implications," *Bell Journal of Economics* 8 (1977): 469, 473. For a general discussion of Hippocratic individualism as well as alternatives to it, see Robert Veatch, *A Theory of Medical Ethics* (New York: Basic Books, 1981), especially chap. 11.

10. See, for example, Renee Fox, *Experiment Perilous* (Glencoe, IL: Free Press, 1959), and Arlene Kaplan Daniels, "The Captive Professional: Bureaucratic Limitations in the Practice of Military Psychiatry," *Journal of Health and Social Behavior* 10 (1969): 255–65.

these competing commitments from the peripheries of medical care, from arguably exceptional situations, to the very center of clinical medicine. In this sense, it is precisely (and paradoxically) the routine character of triage in intensive care that constitutes its novelty.

There is principled resistance to triage among some physicians. There is principled enthusiasm among others. Of the two hospitals included in this study, the resistance is greater at Outerboro, the enthusiasm greater at Countryside. That this difference should exist is, I suspect, largely a consequence of the different tones set by the directors of the two units. As such, the difference is, at least from the point of view of social structural explanation, largely idiosyncratic. However, the difference in the beliefs of physicians in the two units notwithstanding, both Hippocratic individualism and utilitarianism have roots deep in the structure of medical practice. And it is a central contention of this chapter that basic characteristics of intensive care will tend, over the long run, to push physicians away from the former and toward the latter.

Costs and Triage

Intensive care is expensive. By most estimates, a day in a unit costs three or four times as much as a day in a general hospital bed. The high cost of intensive care includes not only the charge for a unit bed (currently on the order of $1,000 a day compared to $500 for a general hospital bed) but also the cost of more frequent blood tests ($20 for each platelet count, $25 for a blood glucose, as much as $100 for a blood culture), X-rays ($100 for an X-ray of the abdomen, as much as $400 for an upper gastrointestinal series), CAT scans ($400), and dialysis (roughly $500 but significantly more at some hospitals).[11] Add all the other various interventions characteristic of units and the totals mount quickly. In one 1982 study of a Los Angeles teaching hospital, Chassin found that, for 489 patients with an average ICU stay of approximately five days, charges averaged $5,698.[12] By 1990, average charges likely more than doubled that figure. At an aggregate level the sums are genuinely staggering. Charges probably exceeded $20 billion dollars annually by the beginning of the 1990s, accounting for over one-seventh of all hospital costs or 1 percent of the total Gross National Product of the United States.

11. Estimated from the United Hospital Fund, *Hospital Rate Directory* (New York: United Hospital Fund of New York, 1986).

12. Mark R. Chassin, "Costs and Outcomes of Medical Intensive Care," *Medical Care* 20 (1982): 165–79.

The costs of intensive care are not, however, evenly distributed over the ICU patient population. For longer admissions and for admissions marked by unusually frequent or complex procedures, costs increase proportionately. Kelly Connors's two months in the Countryside unit generated a bill well in excess of a half-million dollars. In Chassin's study, a subgroup consisting of just over 7 percent of ICU patients accounted for nearly one-third of ICU charges. Moreover, although the results have not been consistent, some research does suggest at least a possibility that the high-cost subgroup of ICU patients includes a disproportionate share of those who do not survive their unit or hospital admission.[13]

In an age of nearly obsessive concern over the costs of health care in general, it is hardly surprising that a concern over the costs of intensive care in particular should lurk behind public policy efforts to develop more systematic strategies of triage. "Considering the level of investment in intensive care and the speed with which it has been rising," Chassin has argued, "it is important to define carefully which patients most benefit from it, the degree to which they benefit and the cost of those additional benefits."[14] Predictive models, then, are the tools with which those patients who contribute most to the costs of intensive care can be identified. Triage, based on those models, is—by implication, if never quite explicitly—the tool with which those costs can be controlled.

Public policy, however, is one thing; clinical practice, quite another. To be sure, the physicians at both Outerboro and Countryside are acutely aware of the cost of intensive care.

One of the Countryside residents had removed the chest tubes from Mr. Hope, a 66-year-old cancer patient who was being kept electively in the unit. John was sarcastic: "Talk about cost containment. You take the tubes out, but you keep someone here five days."

Standing in front of Mr. Trombly's bed in the Outerboro unit, Steve, one of the residents, asked how much a blood gas cost. Another resident answered: forty-five dollars. "Mr. Trombly," Steve went on, "has three sheets of them." The other resident

13. In addition to Chassin, "Costs and Outcomes," see Allan S. Detsky, Steven C. Stricker, Albert G. Mulley, and George E. Thibault, "Prognosis, Survival, and the Expenditure of Hospital Resources for Patients in an Intensive Care Unit," *New England Journal of Medicine* 305 (1981): 667–72; Jeffrey R. Parno, Daniel Teres, Stanley Lemeshow, and Richard Brown, "Hospital Charges and Long-Term Survival of ICU versus Non-ICU Patients," *Critical Care Medicine* 10 (1982): 569–74; David J. Cullen, Roberta Keene, Christine Watenaux, Judith Kunsman, Debra J. Caldera, and Harriet Peterson, "Results, Charges, and Benefits of Intensive Care for Critically Ill Patients: Update 1983," *Critical Care Medicine* 12 (1984): 102–6.
14. Chassin, "Costs and Outcomes," p. 165.

again: "He's over sixty-five. Medicare will pay 80 percent." But Steve went on: "I'm not thinking about the cost to him. Just the cost in general, to the taxpayers, or someone."

Standing in front of Kelly Connors's room at Countryside, her intern noted that she now had a special bed, one that rotated her automatically. "It should," the resident added, "for three hundred dollars a day. . . . We're in the wrong business. We should be in hospital supplies."

Moreover, at least a few physicians are deeply critical of priorities in American medicine, believing that the emphasis on acute interventions has diverted funds more appropriately spent, as one resident put it, on "chronic disease, prophylaxis, prevention." "I really don't care what it costs the hospital," another added,

as much as what it costs the health care system. I'm conscious that everything I do is that two dollars a person that would save people from being blind in Africa. And you should never forget that. . . . I mean it's true and very hypocritical of doctors. Here we are saving lives, sort of, and there are tremendous populations of people that need to be helped and we are not helping them.

These criticisms, however, are rarely translated into clinical decisions. As the very same resident who insisted on his concern for "the tremendous populations . . . that need to be helped" acknowledged only a little later, when "you . . . put someone in the intensive care unit, you have to spend a huge amount of money on them and quibbling over the cost of one antibiotic is unreasonable." Another resident agreed: "Our decisions are based on reversibility of disease and long-term prognosis and viability . . . regardless of the cost." Indeed, aside from an occasional suggestion that a less expensive antibiotic could be substituted for an essentially equivalent, more expensive one, I witnessed, over the course of my entire research, only one instance in which there was even a suggestion that cost was a consideration in a clinical decision: an imputation by one of the Countryside residents that a private physician, associated with a Health Maintenance Organization, wanted his patient moved from the Medical ICU to the Cardiac Care Unit because the charges in the latter were lower. Many physicians at both Countryside and Outerboro believe that cost should be a consideration in intensive care. None believe it is. None practice medicine in a way that would make it so.

At the level of hospital administration, economic considerations may be critical in determining the number of ICU beds available in a given hospital (and, ultimately, in the hospital system as a whole). But triage in the clinical setting is not driven by economic considerations. It is, however, driven by a constant demand for unit beds. Whatever the ultimate implications this de-

mand holds for costs, the demand for beds and cost considerations occupy
very different points in the experience of physicians. While both health care
funds generally and ICU beds in particular are limited resources, the individual physician has far more control over beds than over funds. If, on the
one hand, a doctor saves the hospital—or, for that matter, "society"—one
thousand dollars by denying a patient admission to an intensive care unit or
sending that patient out one day earlier, that doctor has no control over the
savings and no guarantee that those savings will remain in the health care
system. On the other hand, the number of beds in an ICU is fixed, at least
from the perspective of daily care. A bed freed in the ICU, whether by denying an admission or by transferring a patient out, will remain in the system,
available for another, potentially more needy patient. What makes the demand for beds different from economic pressures more generally is that the
allocation of beds is part of a closed system whereas the allocation of economic resources more generally is not.[15]

The contrast between cost considerations and bed pressures helps clarify
the different sources of Hippocratic individualism and a utilitarian ethic. A
"single-minded devotion" to individual patients makes sense in matters of
cost—as a strategy of maximizing the resources available for medical care (a
logic perhaps encouraged by the knowledge that most charges will be picked
up not by individual patients but by either private insurers or the public).
What is given to one patient is not, at least in the short run, taken from
another. In contrast, the pressure for beds encourages a logic of utilitarianism. Because the number of beds is fixed, what is given to one patient is, very
directly, denied another. If the high costs of intensive care require no judgments (or only highly abstract judgments) from physicians about the compar-
ative needs of patients, the demand for beds makes such judgments both
concrete and virtually inevitable.

Bed Pressure

The starting point, then, for any discussion of triage at Outerboro and
Countryside is a simple observation. The units are almost always full or close

15. The argument here draws on Norman Daniels, "Why Saying No to Patients in the
United States Is So Hard," *New England Journal of Medicine* 314 (1986): 1380–83. Daniels's
argument is based on a comparison of medicine in the United States with medicine in Great
Britain. But the intensive care unit re-creates in miniature, and almost uniquely in American
medicine, exactly the closed character of British fixed regional budgets that has made "saying
no" easier for doctors in England than in the United States. See also Aaron and Schwartz,
Painful Prescription.

to it. In the fourteen-bed Outerboro unit, occupancy averaged 93 percent. In the twenty-two-bed Countryside unit (during what the unit director insisted was an unusually slow time), it averaged 84 percent. At Outerboro (as shown in fig. 14.1), of the 114 days for which I have data, the unit was full on 41, had one empty bed on 49, and two empty beds on 17. At Countryside (as shown in fig. 14.2), of the 57 days for which I have data, the unit was full on 11, had one empty bed on 7, and two empty beds on 6. Given that the Outerboro ICU averaged two admissions a day and the Countryside unit (including the surgical service) over four, the pressure to make beds available was almost relentless at both.

In response to this pressure, both Outerboro and Countryside have developed procedures to retain some control over who is admitted to the unit and who is not as well as over who is kept in the unit and who, not. The principles underlying these two types of decisions (about admission to and transfer from intensive care) are very similar. But in practice they are very different and I will describe each in turn.

At both Outerboro and Countryside requests for admission to the units are generated by physicians on the general medical floors or from the Emergency Room. At Outerboro, these requests are directed to a third-year resident who, for a stretch of two weeks at a time, holds the position of medical admitting resident (MAR) for the entire hospital. At Countryside, requests for admission are directed to whichever of the three "intensivists" is the day's triage officer. At Countryside, the intensivist will, especially when the unit is busy, ask the unit resident to assess the patient in question, if only briefly. At

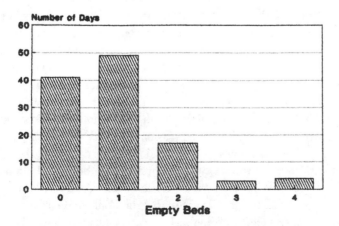

Figure 14.1. Daily number of empty beds, Outerboro.

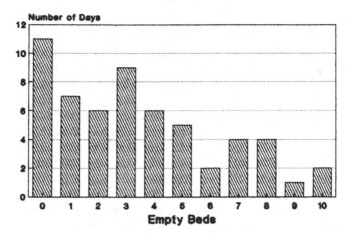

Figure 14.2. Daily number of empty beds, Countryside.

Outerboro, no one from the unit sees the patient before admission. The assignment of responsibility for ICU admission to the MAR or a triage officer is meant, at both hospitals, to detach that decision from primary physicians who might act out of "single-minded devotion" to their own patients. Both systems are meant—altogether explicitly—to encourage a utilitarian ethos. In practice, however, neither system works very well.

The weakness of the system at Outerboro became clear to me when I asked a series of MARs to collect data on patients they were turning down for admission—an effort I abandoned when I realized how rarely they turned down any requests. Over the course of several weeks, four different MARs reported admitting sixty-five patients to either the Intensive Care Unit or the Cardiac Care Unit. In contrast, they reported turning down only four requests for admission. In three of the admissions, the MAR arranged a transfer to the ICU despite reservations that the patient was "not sick enough" to justify the use of a unit bed. In three more admissions, the MAR expressed reservations about a transfer because of the patient's "poor prognosis." In four cases, the admission required "bumping" another patient out of the unit. In fourteen more cases, the admission filled the last bed in the unit.

If the MAR denies requests for admission only occasionally, the ICU physicians themselves deny them even less often. Outerboro ICU physicians do retain some right to refuse admissions, even after patients have been accepted by the MAR. But they exercise this right only in the rarest of circumstances. As one resident explained, "The way I look at it, I've never evaluated a patient before he comes to the unit. We never send people, spies, to make sure a person's sick enough to come in. . . . If a person needs a unit, if we have a bed, then I think it has to be that way." In short, if a physician requests a bed for a patient, that request is usually honored.

I did not repeat the experiment of following the equivalent of the MAR at Countryside, yet it seems unlikely that the triage officers there turned down requests for admission any more frequently than did the MARs at Outerboro. To be sure, the Countryside unit itself retains somewhat more control over admissions than does the Outerboro unit. Because the triage officer is an intensivist and because the unit resident himself or herself evaluates potential admissions, they are occasionally able to "block" what they consider inappropriate admissions. A resident:

I have gone to assess patients in the Emergency Room and assessed patients on the floor whom I felt shouldn't go to the ICU, and then I would call the attending and present the case. And in most instances the patient would not come to the Intensive Care Unit. Sometimes I could find a simple change on the floor that would alleviate their fears or would change the clinical picture. . . . Sometimes it was a problem of the ICU being full. I don't have any problem assessing a patient and saying that in my judgment they shouldn't come here.

Yet the differences between Countryside and Outerboro notwithstanding, neither the triage officer nor the unit resident turned down requests for admission with any great frequency.

The unit was full when I arrived at the hospital in the morning. I asked Ken, who had been triage officer the night before, if he had had to turn anyone away. "No," he answered, "it's the Statue of Liberty." I asked what he meant. He smiled, "What's inscribed on the bottom." ["Give me your tired, your poor . . ."]

An occasional exception aside, then, the restraint in regard to unit admissions depends on the goodwill of physicians on the floors and in the Emergency Room. And when beds are in fact tight, physicians outside the unit may decrease their demands to get patients in. That something of this sort happens at both Countryside and Outerboro seems likely. When the unit is full, requests for admissions decline:

The Countryside ICU was more than full, with twenty-three patients in a unit with nursing staff adequate to cover only twenty-two. I asked John, who had been on duty the night before, if he had had to turn anyone away. "No," he said, "word gets out and people don't call up with marginal requests."

The results of these processes are shown in figure 14.3 in the form of a regression equation plotting the number of admissions over the course of a day by the number of empty beds at the beginning of that day. At Outerboro,

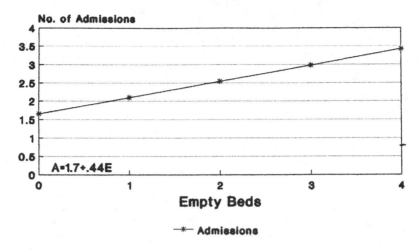

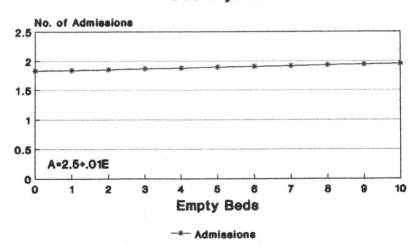

Figure 14.3. Daily admissions by empty beds.

on days that begin with fewer empty beds, there are fewer admissions. On days that begin with more empty beds, there are more admissions. (The same pattern holds only very weakly, if at all, at Countryside.) Despite the weakness of the MAR system, figure 14.3 provides systematic evidence that triage does go on at the point of admission to the Outerboro unit. In contrast, the evidence for triage at the point of admission to the Countryside unit is at best ambiguous.

In decisions to transfer patients out, however, there is no ambiguity. At Outerboro, morning rounds routinely end with a review of which patients should go out and which are "bumps," patients the ICU staff would like to keep but who can be transferred out if beds become tight. At Countryside, a blackboard in one of the nursing stations is set aside for a triage list, constantly updated throughout the day. At both hospitals, final responsibility for transfer decisions rests with an attending, and, at both, the attending consults regularly with the housestaff and nursing staff. Frequently an attending, a house officer, or a nurse will object to the transfer of a particular patient. Occasionally, especially at Outerboro, someone will object to the process of triage in general. But objections notwithstanding, triage does go on.

Moreover, the process is altogether explicit. Consider, first, two discussions—one at Countryside, the other at Outerboro—on days the units were full. In both instances, the lack of empty beds provided a powerful impetus to transfer out patients who, in other circumstances, the ICU physicians would have preferred to keep in the unit a little longer.

Mr. Black, a 56-year-old man with a pulmonary embolus, had been admitted to the Countryside ICU the night before. Although Mr. Black was awake and alert, his private physician had strong reservations about his leaving the unit. But the unit attending saw things differently: "He's got to go out. We need beds." Mr. Black was transferred that afternoon.

Mr. Dewey, a 36-year-old man with active tuberculosis, a four-month cough, and a forty-pound weight loss, was neither intubated nor on pressors, both high-risk interventions which, by Outerboro policy, require the intensive monitoring available only in a unit. Eleven of the twelve unit beds were full. Even before morning rounds had begun, the residents had arranged to transfer Mr. Dewey out of the unit and back to the same ward team that had been caring for him the day before. When this plan was presented to the two attending physicians responsible for the unit, they expressed reservations. One said, "He's the type who'd benefit from being watched." The residents did not disagree, but one explained, "Just in terms of the situation, the CCU [Cardiac Care Unit] is full, with no bumps." The second attending was convinced, although still not happy about the situation: "He's low priority for an ICU bed. The question is whether it's better to go out in the light of day to a team that knows him or in the middle of the night." Mr. Dewey was transferred that afternoon.

The process works the other way as well. When the unit has beds, ICU physicians are inclined to hang on to patients whom, in other circumstances, they would transfer out.

In a discussion of keeping a 68-year-old woman with diabetic ketoacidosis in the Outerboro unit for an additional day, one of the attendings argued, "If you're not pressed for beds, I'd say keep her. . . . If you're pressed for beds, a telemetry unit would be a good place for her to go."

Pete Crawford had been admitted to the Countryside unit with a drug overdose. "Normally," Ken explained, "he wouldn't have come up here, but the unit isn't busy." When an intern suggested that, "if push comes to shove, he can go out tonight," Ken counseled caution: "We've got plenty of beds." Crawford stayed the night.

At the end of a discussion of Mr. Grant, a 91-year-old man recovering from sepsis, one attending asked the residents, "In terms of sending him out, what are your plans?" A resident answered, "We don't want to send him out." A second resident explained, "In terms of beds, we haven't been pressured." The attending agreed: "Looking over there I see lots of white sheets [meaning empty beds]. We don't have to be in a hurry. . . . Remember that an ICU doesn't have to be for people on the brink of death."

Figure 14.4 shows the results of this process in a regression equation plotting the average length of unit stay of discharged patients by the number of empty beds on the day of their discharge. At both Outerboro and Countryside, patients are discharged after shorter unit stays when there are fewer empty beds. When there are more empty beds, they are discharged after longer unit stays. In short, there is strong evidence that, at both hospitals, physicians discharge and retain patients depending on the availability of beds.

To some of the unit physicians, these processes and the constant pressure to triage are easy to explain. There are too many sick patients and not enough unit beds. But this is too easy. The number of beds in the unit is fixed, at least in the short run. But the number of sick patients is not. While the supply of beds is fixed, the demand for those beds is highly flexible, contracting when beds are scarce, expanding when they are plentiful.

A study conducted at Massachusetts General Hospital by Daniel Singer and his associates supports this observation. When a nursing shortage forced Massachusetts General to reduce its ICU beds from eighteen to between eight and fourteen, Singer found that the proportion of patients admitted only for monitoring decreased precipitously and the proportion admitted for major interventions increased correspondingly.[16] While Singer was most

16. Daniel Singer, Phyllis Carr, Albert Mulley, and George Thibault, "Rationing Intensive Care—Physician Responses to a Resource Shortage," *New England Journal of Medicine* 309

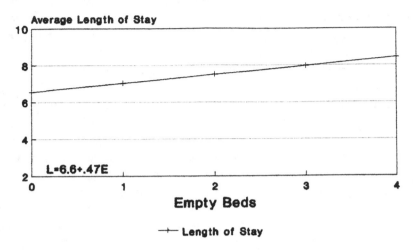

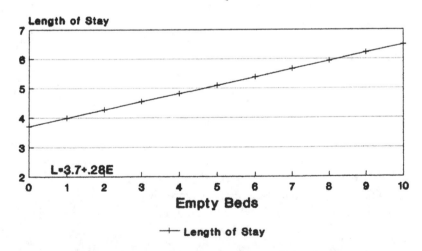

Figure 14.4. Average length of stay of discharges by empty beds.

concerned to point out that physicians apply more stringent criteria for admission to and retention in an ICU when fewer beds are available, we might as easily point out that they apply less stringent criteria when more beds are available. Put simply, physicians' working concept of the acuity of illness requiring intensive care varies with the availability of beds.

The pressure for beds, then, is not simply a function of the number of patients who, in some objective sense, need intensive care. While there are some "absolute" indications for ICUs—of which the most important is intensive nursing care on a ventilator—there are often insufficient patients with such indications to fill the units. As a result, the units are filled with patients who might benefit from some aspect of intensive care, even if they do not absolutely require it. They are in intensive care because their physicians want them to receive optimal medical care. But the appeals of intensive care—the higher ratio of nursing staff to patients, the attentiveness of housestaff, the greater availability of various equipment—are sufficient to ensure that, for all practical purposes, there will always be patients who could benefit. Thus, the problem for physicians is not determining who needs intensive care and who does not on the basis of absolute indications. In the very logic of the way demand is generated for medical care, the problem is rather to determine priorities among patients whose physicians' appetite for intensive care is insatiable. As long as there is a hierarchy of care in medicine, as long as ICUs are at or near the top of that hierarchy, and as long as the number of ICU beds is finite (a condition likely to remain the case for some time to come), there will be pressure to fill those beds. And, as long as there is pressure to fill those beds, triage is inevitable.

Principles

There is surprisingly little disagreement among the intensive care doctors at either Outerboro or Countryside (or, for that matter, between the two hospitals) over the principles of triage. Moreover, the principles of triage roughly parallel criteria used in deciding how aggressively to treat.

Criteria of social worth, while raised more often than in decisions to limit

---

(1983): 1155–60. See also Michael J. Strauss, James P. LoGerfo, James Yeltatzie, Nancy Temkin, and Leonard D. Hudson, "Rationing of Intensive Care Unit Services: An Everyday Occurrence," *Journal of the American Medical Association* 255 (1986): 1143–46. For a different view, see Mark A. Kelley, Diane C. Nachamkin, Jose J. Escarce, Neil I. Goldfarb, Paul N. Lanken, and Sankey V. Williams, "Expansion of the Medical Intensive Care Unit: Clinical Consequences in a Large Urban Hospital," *Critical Care Medicine* 18 (1990): 945–49.

treatment, are nonetheless self-consciously ignored. Most of the housestaff and a few of the attendings are anything but shy about judging what they imagine to be the contributions to society that some of their patients are making. Some are even prepared to suggest that particularly difficult patients should not be admitted to the unit. But such suggestions are not entirely serious.

Mr. Santana, a 35-year-old intravenous drug user and diabetic, had been admitted to the Countryside ICU for management of his diabetic ketoacidosis. Grant, Santana's intern, described him: "Here's a guy who was on [the ward], who was eating ice cream and was refusing to take his insulin. He's an idiot." Ken asked what his home life was like, and the resident answered: "Terrible. He's an IVDA [intravenous drug abuser]." "What," Ken asked, "would you do with this type of patient population, not treat him?" Grant answered simply: "Institutionalize him." Santana stayed in the unit until his diabetic crisis had passed.

Suggestions to triage patients of questioned social worth are, then, a type of social criticism—a sort of perverse utopianism, an imagination of a world in which all patients are not only fine citizens, but also grateful and compliant. Such suggestions are not intended to guide actual clinical decisions. Indeed, in the few instances in which one or another physician seems to propose social worth seriously as a criterion in a triage decision, the proposal is quickly rejected.

As in decisions to limit treatment, physicians treat the age of patients ambivalently. All else being equal, or nearly so, the ICU doctors give preference to younger patients over older ones.

When one of the Outerboro residents suggested sending out Mrs. Viscuso, a young woman in the unit with complications following her pregnancy, now awake and alert and off the respirator, Dennis objected strenuously. "She's young. She's 29 and vibrant. Do you want to get another 80-year-old with a fractured hip?"

Mr. Gallo, a 93-year-old man with mild heart disease, was stable after his admission to the Countryside ICU. A nurse reported that "the family's very nervous about him going out to the floor. They're worried that, just because of his age, he won't get good care on the floor." Smiling, John answered, "Tell them we don't usually let 90-year-olds in."

A Countryside resident made the logic explicit: someone who is younger is "much more deserving of resources. . . . There are [two patients] competing for the same resources. You can say, medically, the 25-year-old patient has more of a chance."

Of course, all else is rarely equal and both units treat many older patients. The average age of patients is 58 at Outerboro and 57 at Countryside. Moreover, patients over 65 typically stay in the units longer than do younger ones (an average of 7.1 days at Outerboro compared to 6.3 days for younger patients, and an average of 5.1 at Countryside compared to 3.7). Because older patients are often significantly sicker than younger ones, this hardly constitutes evidence that older patients are treated in the same way as younger ones, *given the same acuity of illness.* It is, however, evidence that—their preferences notwithstanding—ICU physicians neither systematically exclude older patients from the units nor rush them out once admitted.

Ignoring costs and rejecting both social worth and (for the most part) age as criteria for triage, the physicians at both Outerboro and Countryside want patients who will benefit from the unit's (and their own) efforts. Most important, they want to admit and retain patients whose conditions they believe are remediable. John, an enthusiast of prediction models, is entirely explicit on this point:

I think the standard of care should be appropriateness of medical care. There may be other issues involved, but I think that ought to be one of the standards. It is clear, given a constellation of diseases, that a patient isn't going to recover. For large numbers of patients with that same constellation of disease, of severity, then that patient shouldn't be treated. It's a waste of a resource.

Similar views are echoed routinely and insistently by virtually all the house-staff and attendings at both Countryside and Outerboro. An attending:

What happens with allocation and resources is that, once someone that is very sick gets into the unit, . . . you find out that you can't help them. And then you can't get them out of the unit. That is where the major allocation problem is. We have these long-term patients whose admission was appropriate at the time, but later data indicate that they have no reversible disease and are going to require respirator therapy or some other ICU type of support. And they're taking up a bed that some person with a more acute, more quickly reversible problem . . . could use.

In short, physicians at both Outerboro and Countryside espouse principles of medical utility.

Remediability, as discussed in chapter 10, consists not just of the likelihood of physiological survival but also of the likelihood of recovering mental capacities.

Two weeks after the cardiac arrest of Kelly Connors, whose case was reported at the beginning of this chapter, her resident reported that her respiration was improving. "It's actually kind of unfortunate. She's going to be physiologically better and then brain dead." When one of the attendings corrected him, pointing out that Kelly was far from brain dead, the resident went on: "No, but she's not going to be applying for any Rhodes scholarships. The unfortunate thing is her family wants her alive and they don't care if she's low functioning." No one disagreed, and a little later Ken added, "I'd have no problem with treating her on the floor. But this is a waste of resources."

Moreover, physicians evaluate triage decisions on criteria of short-term, rather than long-term, remedy—in particular, against the possibility of successful discharge from the unit and the hospital. None of the physicians at either hospital objects to devoting a bed to a cancer patient with an acute, reversible condition—even if that patient's long-term prognosis is grim. Few object to admitting and retaining AIDS patients, at least for a first episode of the pneumonia that characterizes that disease.

Roger Sherman had been admitted to the Outerboro ICU with a confirmed diagnosis of AIDS. Faced with the usual shortage of beds, one of the residents ranked his priority against Ortiz, a man with a severe gastrointestinal bleed. "I'd send out Sherman before Ortiz because Sherman has a limited prognosis." But Dennis disagreed: "He could walk out and be hit by a car. So don't talk about that. It's a question of what we can do."

The principle is similar to that applied to old patients. Although physicians prefer patients with potentially long lives ahead of them, they treat any patient with the possibility of leaving the hospital, even one with what seems likely to be a short life span, as warranting admission.

Finally, in both units admissions and discharges are based on capabilities specific to the ICU, as determined by the availability of staff and equipment and by hospital policy. Although in both hospitals there are provisions for providing some ventilator support outside the unit, in neither does that support go beyond its simplest forms. Thus, in both units preference is given for admission and retention to patients who require ventilator support. "The attendings always joke," an Outerboro resident told me, "that, 'God forbid, you shouldn't be intubated when you're in a unit.' Because it means you'll be bumped out in two hours." In neither hospital does a Do Not Resuscitate order disqualify a patient from admission to the unit, although in each the patient must be able to benefit from some aspect of intensive care other than its capacity for quick responses to cardiac and respiratory arrests. And in both units patients are sometimes admitted and retained for no reason other than that they require the intensive nursing care available only in ICUs.

In short, in both units the physicians are committed to conducting triage on principles of medical utility. There may be frequent and intense disagreements about the application of these principles, in particular as to which patient will benefit more from the unit. But as to the principles themselves there is little disagreement. Neither is there a great deal in these principles that most medical ethicists would object to—with the possible exception of the bias toward younger patients. Nor is there a great deal that devotees of predictive models would object to—except, perhaps, to wish that judgments of benefit were based on sounder scientific research.

Principles, however, are one thing. Practice is another. Indeed, in many of the incidents I have just cited, the principle of medical utility is articulated only in response to its frequent violation. While the structure of intensive care medicine encourages the adoption of a utilitarian ethos in general, that ethos is applied unevenly. Some circumstances are exempted from an otherwise standard calculation of benefits. These exemptions are not distributed randomly across the patient population. Rather, the distribution of these exemptions is socially structured in such a way as to create systematic biases in the application of medical utility to triage.

Practices

Three factors, in particular, interfere with the evenhanded application of principles of medical utility. The first is a general bias toward excluding patients who are "not sick enough" in favor of admitting and retaining patients who are "too sick"; the second, an attachment to some (but not all) families; the third, the continued presence in intensive care of private physicians alongside interns, residents, and ICU staff.

In the first instance, compare the practice of triage in intensive care with battlefield practice. Battlefield triage implies a clear mandate: bypass both those patients whose conditions are not sufficiently acute to need immediate attention and those patients whose conditions are too acute to benefit from any medical attention in favor of those who will benefit most. It is a simple principle of medical utility. Civilian triage, at least as it is practiced in the intensive care units at Outerboro and Countryside, is different. While those patients whose conditions are not sufficiently acute to warrant unit care are, indeed, bypassed, there is frequent reluctance to bypass those whose conditions are too acute.

This reluctance can be seen, in part, at the point of admission to the unit. In the survey I conducted of Outerboro MAR admitting practices, all four of the requests for admission that the MARs reported denying were on grounds that the patient was "not sick enough." In not a single instance did they report turning down a request for admission because the patient was "too sick."

The reluctance to exclude patients who are too sick to be helped by the ICU is even more evident in decisions about retention and discharge. In earlier chapters, I discussed at great length the reasons physicians often continue to treat dying patients. It suffices here to point out the implications of that reluctance for triage. In particular, at neither hospital do the ICU physicians easily remove support from respirator-dependent patients, even from those who are comatose and without significant chance of recovery. At Countryside, a few special circumstances aside, they will remove respirators only with the agreement of the family. As in the case of Kelly Connors, that agreement is not always forthcoming. At Outerboro, they will remove respirators only in very rare circumstances, if at all. In the case of Scranton Haskell they removed the respirator only after they had determined that Haskell could survive without it, at least in the short run.

What makes these considerations significant for triage, however, is not simply the reluctance of physicians to discontinue respirator support. It is that reluctance in combination with the scarcity of locations in which such support can be offered outside the ICU. Few nurses outside the units have either the time or the skills necessary to care for respirator-dependent patients. At Outerboro, hospital policy bars respirator-dependent patients from the general medical floors. Although there is a four-bed Respirator Room, intended as a step-down unit, it is usually filled (as was the case with Haskell). At Countryside, hospital policy does permit the floors to accept patients on respirators but with the stipulation that respiratory settings cannot be adjusted after admission to the floor. The step-down unit there works even less well than the one at Outerboro.

The extent of the dilemma, particularly at Outerboro, can hardly be overestimated, for respirator-dependent patients with poor prognoses are, at least in that setting, unusually heavy users of ICU beds. At Countryside, all ten of the longest ICU stays, an average of twenty-three days each, were accounted for by respirator-dependent patients, six of whom died without leaving the hospital. At Outerboro, nineteen of the twenty patients with the longest unit stays, an average of forty-nine days each, were respirator dependent and sixteen of the nineteen died without leaving the hospital. Even at Countryside, the situation is sometimes difficult:

You are in a tight situation all the time. Who do you send out first? You often send out the patient who is not on a ventilator, who really is being pushed out because he is not on hardware, so to speak. And the one who winds up staying in the unit is the patient having a downhill climb, becoming unsalvageable.

At Outerboro, it is even more difficult. I had asked one of the residents if there were ever times when a bed could not be found for a patient who needed the ICU. "All the time," he answered, largely because we're filled with dead patients. A number of times you have a GI bleeder on the floor or somebody with ketoacidosis, or any of the number of diseases that are very well handled in the intensive care unit, . . . who should be in the Medical ICU. There's a large number of times that there are no beds and twelve intubated patients, nine of whom are certainly going to die.

Even allowing for exaggeration, this is a situation that can in no way be confused with the evenhanded application of medical utility.

The general bias toward retaining patients whose conditions are too acute to benefit from intensive care—patients who are "too sick"—is not the result of a failure to articulate clear or consensual ethical principles. To the contrary, there is general and explicit agreement, at least among the physicians at Outerboro and Countryside, that such patients receive far too much preference for a scarce resource. Neither can the bias be attributed to any failure of predictive models. The ICU physicians have little difficulty identifying many of the respirator-dependent patients whose prognoses are grim. Rather, the bias results, in part, from a failure of organization—from the unwillingness or inability of hospital administrators to provide adequate step-down units. Even more, it results from a failure of authority—from the inability of physicians to convince families to hold back on aggressive efforts and from their reluctance (whether from genuine ethical scruples or from fear of legal consequences) to withdraw treatment.

The bias toward patients who are "too sick" interferes with the application of principles of medical utility, but it does not imply a movement back toward Hippocratic individualism. In contrast, an attachment to families and the continued presence of private physicians in intensive care both interfere with utilitarian principles and restore aspects of Hippocratic individualism—albeit in a highly particularistic form.

If intensive care patients themselves, typically unable to speak and often comatose, rarely form significant relationships with the staff physicians who are caring for them, their husbands, wives, children, and parents can. Indeed, the families of patients assume significance in intensive care precisely to the degree that the patients themselves are unresponsive. Recalling one case, an Outerboro resident remembered:

His wife was there every day. This woman was just very nice. There was something, it was moving, about her just sitting there day in and day out. So some of [the time], once you've spoken to a family member, then the whole relationship changes. You know them and they know you. . . . Some people don't like to talk to families but I actually do. In the unit, it's the only kind of personal interaction you have since the patient is completely out of it.

An attachment to a family often exercises a powerful force. Certainly it did in the cases of both Kelly Connors and Scranton Haskell, with which I began this chapter.

With Connors, an attachment to her family may have diminished Ken's ability to distance himself from the case. Her family, particularly her father and fiancé, were in the unit's waiting room day and night. They greeted the unit physicians and nurses each morning with a zeal and optimism remarkable under the trying circumstances in which they found themselves. As Ken—usually insistently hard-boiled—himself confessed to the housestaff before finally threatening to withdraw from the case, "I had dinner with a friend of mine last night. We had a long talk, and I realized I wasn't thinking clearly. I've been manipulated by the family. I wasn't thinking as a physician. I was influenced too much by my feelings for the father."

In Haskell's case, Dennis came to think of the family itself as the patient. In his case, when most of the unit residents were eager to transfer him, Dennis posed the issue very differently: "Aren't we waiting until we can treat the wife? . . . She's the one who's awake and walking around." Discussing the case later, one of the residents concurred:

I think it was a good thing to treat the wife. When we get to this point, where we get patients who are comatose and have no idea of what's going on, then it is true that a lot of our commitment kind of shifts: less emphasis on the patient, more emphasis on the family. It was a good thing to prepare the wife.

It is, perhaps, hard to criticize either Ken or Dennis for the positions they took. Yet concern for families, however well intentioned, departs significantly from a principle of medical utility. Moreover, it introduces a systematic bias toward those patients with families, those whose families are frequent visitors to the unit, and, perhaps, those whose families the physicians find appealing. Such a bias is no more than a slight crack in the application of medical utility to triage, but it is a crack through which criteria of social worth have begun to sneak back in.

If an attachment to families puts a slight crack in the application of medical utility, the continued presence in the ICU of private physicians drives it wider. The units at both Outerboro and Countryside are "classless" in the sense that they admit Medicaid patients and patients with no medical insurance of any kind as well as patients with private insurance. Both admit patients with private physicians as well as those without. At both units patients are assigned to beds with studied indifference as to whether their physicians are the most senior privates or the newest of housestaff. Yet the influence of privates remains. At Outerboro, official policy is that the unit staff assumes primary responsibility for all patients, even those with private physicians. Although the unit physicians take this responsibility very seriously, many private physicians continue to follow their patients after an intensive care admission and, in some instances, continue to play an active role in their care. At Countryside, the influence of private physicians is even stronger. Although some privates turn care over to the intensivists and the housestaff, others (to the near inevitable annoyance of the housestaff) continue to direct the care of their patients themselves, sometimes calling in the intensivists as consultants and sometimes almost entirely on their own.

For private physicians to set a course of treatment for their patients or to reserve to themselves critical decisions about those patients is, of course, hardly a matter to comment on. It is simply standard practice in American medicine. Neither should it be surprising that private physicians often have deep commitments to their patients. Indeed, unit physicians frequently defer to privates because the privates have established long-term relationships of precisely the sort that is typically missing in intensive care. What is to the point, however, is that the commitment of private physicians to their patients interferes with the otherwise evenhanded application of the principles of medical utility.

After the presentation of Mrs. Winters, a patient with metastatic cancer, I asked one of the Outerboro residents what her chances were for survival. He answered, "None. There's no way she'll ever get out of the hospital. It's an abuse of the unit and the patient." I asked how she got into the unit: "Her attending wanted her in." I asked if anyone had objected: "We asked multiple times, but if you've got an advocate, that's it." Mrs. Winters stayed in the unit for over a week.

Mr. Herman had been admitted to the Countryside ICU with end stage pulmonary fibrosis. John was not convinced he should have been admitted at all. "My understanding is that patients with end stage pulmonary fibrosis go to hospice care. We want to avoid intubation. . . . Dr. Jerome [Herman's private] has to convince us why this man has to stay in the ICU." Apparently Dr. Jerome succeeded: Mr. Herman stayed in the ICU two more days.

On morning rounds at Outerboro, the attending was puzzled that Mrs. Russo was still in the unit: "This is the lady who didn't really arrest. Why is she still here?" The resident: "Nancy [her private physician] wanted her here for observations." The attending: "We've done worse things. Okay."

On the third day of her admission to the Countryside ICU, Larry, her intern, had successfully extubated Mrs. Cohen and already written a transfer note. But her private physician expressed reservations. His terse note in the chart read simply: "Continued observation in the ICU seems appropriate." Mrs. Cohen stayed in the unit two more days.

The ability of private physicians to influence triage decisions can be explained, in part, by their location in the hospital's hierarchy of prestige and authority. Sometimes, one Outerboro resident acknowledged, admission decisions "can get very, very political and you have nothing to say about it and accept the patient." More fundamental, though, than differences in the authority of private physicians and housestaff, than differences in "clout," is a difference between the structure of private practice and the structure of a residency, internship, or staff position.

Triage raises general questions about the character and sources of physicians' commitments to individual patients. These are questions more often asked in the opposite direction, in terms of patients' commitment to individual physicians as represented in the large literature on compliance with medical regimens and doctor shopping.[17] Yet, if we take seriously the notion that the doctor-patient relationship is reciprocal, these questions are equally important to ask of physicians in regard to patients.

It is among the most consistent findings of social science applied to medicine—indeed, almost a platitude—that the commitment of patients to individual physicians depends on the quality of doctor-patient interactions. Patients will comply more readily with, return more regularly to, and express a higher level of diffuse satisfaction for those physicians they perceive as caring and concerned. Less often recognized, though, is that the reciprocal commitment of physicians to individual patients depends on parallel considerations. Physicians may not need reassurance that their patients are concerned or caring. But their satisfaction with medical practice may well depend on a perception that their patients understand and appreciate their efforts. This is a satisfaction, as much as for patients, which emerges from the quality of doctor-patient interactions.

Yet intensive care, at Outerboro, Countryside, and elsewhere, is marked, perhaps above all, by a severe attenuation of the doctor-patient relationship, especially when the doctor in question is an intern, resident, or intensivist rather than a private physician. At its core, a relationship, especially a committed relationship, is something which extends over time, something which has not only a present but also a past and a future. However, in the intensive

---

17. See, for a general review of this literature, Bonnie L. Svarstad, "Patient-Practitioner Relationships and Compliance with Prescribed Medical Regimens," in Linda H. Aiken and David Mechanic, eds., *Applications of Social Science to Clinical Medicine and Health Policy*, pp. 438–59 (New Brunswick, NJ: Rutgers University Press, 1986). Questions similar to the ones I am raising here can be found in Raymond Duff and August Hollingshead, *Sickness and Society* (New York: Harper & Row, 1968), especially chap. 8.

care unit—as I argued in greater detail in part I—neither the patient's past nor the patient's future is accessible to the staff physician charged with the patient's care.

Faced with acutely ill patients, nearly one-quarter of whom die without leaving the unit and nearly one-half of whom die without leaving the hospital, ICU physicians fear investing too much—whether emotion or effort—in any one patient. Confronting the limits of medicine, they turn away from a commitment to patients and toward those colleagues who share an understanding of those limits.

If, in private practice, commitment to the individual patient emerges out of a long and continuing relationship, out of the patient's expressions of gratitude for the doctor's efforts, out of a dense set of expression and exchange, all this is missing in intensive care. Occasional exceptions aside (exceptions of the sort that result in attachments to a few families), all that remains are abstract values stressing the priority of individual patients. These values are themselves powerful forces. But no longer rooted in concrete relationship with particular patients, they become vulnerable to conflicting values and counterpressures.

If commitment to individual patients emerges out of the concrete relationships between doctors and patients, so, too, does the commitment to freeing beds emerge out of concrete relationships among physicians. For the housestaff, in particular, the pressure to keep ICU beds available is the specific expression of a general obligation to other residents and interns. In the first instance, "blocking" ICU beds may result in more work for the very people the house officer has trained with and often sees as close friends:

If there were no bed available and there were an arrest, it means the patient needs to be taken care of on the floor by the housestaff. That really means that . . . one of the members of the housestaff is not able to leave that patient and has to ambubag [in effect, ventilate by hand rather than with a respirator] the patient on the floor, which may be hours. The problem is that the turnover of ICU beds happens very slowly. . . . They stand at bedside with the patients. That means that they're pulled away from their other duties. I think that that's not acceptable, when that house officer is responsible for maybe ten or fifteen other patients and usually is pressed for time anyway.

Even more, the failure to open a bed by transferring a patient out in the face of an urgent call from a colleague implies a lack of trust. A resident:

Some of your decisions are based on who is calling you. Someone calls you who you don't really trust—there are just certain people in the program who are out to lunch— and they call you with a unit admission that sounds borderline, you may actually ask the MAR to evaluate the patient. . . . But that is really the minority of cases. Most of the time you take their word for it.

Because they rotate through the wards and private services as well as through the unit, the housestaff, at both Countryside and Outerboro, empathize with the physicians who are requesting admissions. Even more, they understand that they are part of a system of reciprocity.

The people who have decided to put them in the unit have had a hard enough time struggling with that decision and they know the patient and I can't make that job any worse for them. . . . I will help them decide. But I don't think that I can do more than that. I don't think it's fair to the person who is clearly struggling with the same thing that I would be struggling with if I were in his place. I don't expect somebody to give me a hard time if I send somebody to the unit.

The concern for reciprocity is even more intense when the request for an admission comes from another house officer rather than from a private physician:

I've never attempted to keep anyone out because, particularly somebody coming from the floor, there's housestaff taking care of them. They've done the best they can, and they feel this person should come. . . . I'm really not going to try to tell them that they should try harder. People have done that to me when I've been on the wards and I really hate that. . . . I generally don't try to block admission.

Thus, a willingness to triage patients becomes the very currency with which the solidarity of housestaff is purchased. Knowing that their situations may be reversed soon enough, at the end of their rotations, one resident cannot easily deny the urgent request of another resident for a unit bed. Obligations to patients become a matter not of the relationship of individual physicians to individual patients but of the housestaff to each other and of the housestaff as a whole to a patient population as a whole. In this sense, the commitment to individual patients does not compete with commitment to abstract, potential patients but with commitments to other physicians who are friends and colleagues as well as indispensable allies in managing the stresses of training in internal medicine.

Housestaff outside the unit, no less than private physicians, can and do act as advocates for a patient's admission to the unit. However, because residents are bound to other housestaff by a web of mutual obligations, they are less likely to press their requests for admissions against the objections of other housestaff. In contrast, the private physician, located primarily in an office-based practice and thus less concerned with the goodwill of housestaff, is freer to insist on the admission or retention of a patient even against objections. Where the housestaff's obligation to a patient is part of a collective responsibility, the private physician's is individual. Where the housestaff's location in the medical division of labor encourages attention to other physicians and, thus, to other physicians' patients, the private physician's location systematically discourages such attention.[18]

Both housestaff (or intensivists) and private physicians may act on the basis of consistent principles. But because their principles are different—utilitarian among housestaff, those of Hippocratic individualism among privates—the aggregate result is inconsistent. Insofar as middle-class and wealthy patients are likelier to have private physicians and poor patients are likelier to depend on housestaff, the uneven distribution of advocacy over the patient population reintroduces class distinctions even into the "classless" setting of intensive care.

A bias toward retaining dying patients, attachments to families, and the influence of private physicians are all sources of exemptions from the principle of medical utility. Attachments to families and the influence of privates may also be understood as a recrudescence of Hippocratic individualism in a setting otherwise dominated by a utilitarian ethos. But Hippocratic individualism applied to some patients and some circumstances is far different in its consequences from Hippocratic individualism applied to all patients in all circumstances. In intensive care, Hippocratic individualism becomes the basis for objections to triage in particular cases but not to triage in general. But in the context of a medical setting in which beds are scarce, exemptions from triage are themselves incorporated into the very system from which they at first seem exempted. Retaining one patient in the ICU, for whatever reason, implies denying admission to another. Thus, in the context of intensive care, Hippocratic individualism becomes the source not of high ethical principles but of irrationalities and systematic, socially structured biases.

The End of Advocacy?

Notions of Hippocratic individualism have been central to the ideology of American medicine for at least a century. It is on grounds of the essentially dyadic character of the doctor-patient relationship that physicians have resisted third-party payments, group medical practices, and government regulations. Moreover, it is on grounds of advocacy that physicians have asked

18. For a discussion of the social structures that encourage primary loyalty to the patient rather than to the profession, see Eliot Freidson, *Patients' Views of Medical Practice* (New York: Russell Sage, 1961).

for, and for the most part received, the trust of their patients. The practice of triage does not eliminate these claims. It does weaken them.

My findings in two intensive care units, no matter how thoroughly studied, are not, of course, representative in any statistical sense. I would not want to—nor could I—generalize from the findings reported here to any statement about the *distribution* of Hippocratic individualism or a utilitarian ethos in American medicine. Nonetheless, my findings are representative in the more restricted sense that they speak to the unfolding of a logic of medical care. This logic does not tell us how frequently physicians face the dilemmas posed by a scarcity of resources. It does tell us a great deal about how they will respond to such dilemmas and why they will respond in the ways they do.

Although the comparison might make some physicians uneasy, the doctor-patient relationship has, in certain respects, paralleled that of lawyer and client. Like the lawyer, the doctor has acted as a single-minded advocate for the patient. However, unlike the lawyer, for whom advocacy implies conflict with other lawyers' clients, doctors have rarely had to face situations in which their advocacy has conflicted with other doctors' patients. In a sense, doctors have been able to have their cake and eat it too. They have been able to claim both that they are advocates of individual patients and that, in the course of advocating for individual patients, they are contributing to an aggregation of optimal medical outcomes for all patients.

A scarcity of resources changes all that. Because the questions posed by a scarcity of resources are still novel to American medicine, the answers to those questions are poorly institutionalized. Unlike lawyers, whose commitment to their equivalent of Hippocratic individualism is supported by the full weight of the American legal system, doctors face a genuine dilemma between two competing principles. Unlike lawyers, doctors have a choice. But that choice is itself socially structured.

A scarcity of resources alone does not account for the decline of Hippocratic individualism in intensive care. Rather, the scarcity of beds accounts for only some of the movement toward utilitarian principles. If physicians continued to have strong commitments to individual patients, they would likely experience considerably more tension between such principles and the "single-minded devotion" to particular patients. The more or less thorough triumph of a utilitarian ethic over Hippocratic individualism in intensive care can be accounted for, then, by a scarcity of resources only when placed in the context of an attenuated relationship between doctor and patient.

In looking beyond intensive care, it is not enough to say that resources are also limited in Health Maintenance Organizations or in transplant programs or even, more generally, by the advent of prospective payment systems. We also have to know how HMOs or transplant programs or prospective payment systems actually affect the doctor-patient relationship and how they affect the web of obligations among physicians themselves. Put somewhat differently, the rise of a utilitarian ethic may have less to do with a scarcity of resources than with the social structure of medical care in which that scarcity occurs.

Commitments to individual patients do not disappear in intensive care, nor are they likely to disappear in American medicine more generally. In the extraordinary patchwork of private practices, residencies, and hospital appointments as well as professional norms, public policy, and legal regulation, all with interlocking and overlapping claims, that makes up the American medical system, no single set of principles is likely to be applied with anything approaching consistency. Yet the practice of triage in intensive care, based on utilitarian principles, introduces something genuinely novel. Triage challenges the most fundamental assumptions of the doctor-patient relationship. Most important, it challenges the notion that physicians will act, not just usually but in all situations, with single-minded devotion to the best interests of each individual patient. If, in the past, physicians have been able to claim that advocacy is consistent with optimal aggregate outcomes, that a commitment to individual patients is consistent with a commitment to patients in general, the practice of triage makes the tension between those competing commitments palpable.

15

Medicine's Two Cultures

Everything has changed. Nothing has changed. Patients' rights have triumphed. Patients' rights have failed. The authority of physicians has vanished. The authority of physicians is intact.

The argument of this book, I fear, may seem to some a series of paradoxes or, worse, contradictions. How can I argue that rights have triumphed and, at the same time, that they have failed, that physicians have been stripped of their authority (and, to some degree, abandoned it) and that they continue to make decisions for patients and their families? Both sides of the argument are, I think, accurate—but partial. The difficulty is in specifying the ways and situations in which each side applies.

How Patients' Rights Have Triumphed

On the face of it, the argument is easy to make. Certainly, clinical decisions in medicine are more heavily regulated now than they were ten years ago, let alone twenty, even leaving aside the massive regulation that has accompanied increased financial stringency. At the core of this new regulation is the doctrine of informed consent. For informed consent has required physicians to invite a type of participation from their patients that was, if not unimaginable, strikingly rare as recently as the 1960s. The extension of informed consent to decisions about termination of treatment—whether in court decisions from Quinlan through to Cruzan, in legislation, or in hospital procedures for writing Do Not Resuscitate orders—has only intensified this trend.

It is altogether to the point in this respect that court cases in matters of medical ethics have paid only scant attention to the interests of physicians. While, for example, the Quinlan court did nod briefly in the direction of maintaining the "integrity of the medical profession," the case nonetheless turned on a question of whether informed consent extended to a right to refuse potentially life-prolonging treatments, an entirely patient-centered question. Similarly, the Cruzan case turned on a question of how best to safeguard informed consent—whether through a surrogate decision or "clear and convincing" evidence of the patient's own wishes. In neither case did the court so much as consider the possibility of physicians' making a determination independent of the patient's wishes.

Not least, physicians themselves seem to have accepted many of the precepts of medical ethics. Most important, many physicians now profess their allegiance to principles of patient autonomy, a value for the most part alien to the long tradition of medical thought. As I have suggested in a number of chapters, the evidence of various surveys, both national and local, as well as my own research suggests that physicians frequently endorse patients' rights to make choices bearing on their own treatment, sometimes with even more enthusiasm than do patients themselves.

On the face of it, patients' rights have triumphed. Yet to leave things at face value would clearly be a mistake.

How Patients' Rights Have Failed

The opposite argument is made just as easily. As I have argued at some length in earlier chapters, much of the legal regulation of medicine simply fails to accomplish what it has set out to do. Whatever the law says, in the absence of effective mechanisms of enforcement, it remains for physicians to apply the law in particular cases. Yet, as I have suggested, although physicians often complain about the law, they know little of its details and often ignore its mandates. In the case of informed consent, both my research and others' suggest that the legal requirement is typically little more than a formality. Not only does the type of decision required by law misrepresent the types of decisions that are made in medicine, but most questions about consent are formulated by physicians in such a way as to induce the kinds of answers physicians want. Moreover, even in the occasional instances in which patients do withhold consent from procedures physicians wish to initiate, physicians often proceed on their own inclinations.

The same considerations bear even more strongly on decisions to limit treatment. In many instances, both court decisions and administrative procedures are simply irrelevant to the issues at hand. Addressed primarily to situations in which patients or families want to withdraw or withhold treatment over the objections of hospital administrators or state officials, most court decisions have ignored the more frequent tension between physicians who want to limit treatment and families who want to "do everything." Similarly, formal Do Not Resuscitate procedures, in their virtually exclusive focus on cardiopulmonary resuscitation, ignore a wide range of treatment choices that are often far more decisive than CPR itself. As a result, despite the apparent density of regulation, most decisions about terminating treatment still take place in a realm of murky legality, filled with ambiguity, open to interpretation and reinterpretation.

This argument also suggests a somewhat different reading of many of the landmark court cases, particularly Quinlan and Cruzan. As has been often noted, Quinlan, whose case is usually and rightly taken as a landmark in the "right to die," lived for over a decade following the court's decision. In contrast, Cruzan, whose case was widely interpreted as restricting families' abilities to terminate treatment, died within a year of the Supreme Court's decision. These outcomes are typically treated as curious ironies, something to be remarked on in passing before getting on to the important business of enunciating the principles underlying the courts' decisions. But they are something more. They are themselves testimony to the irrelevance of the courts and the courts' principles to what actually happens in the course of medical treatment.

We may go further. Although courts, state law, and hospital policies are all virtually unanimous in their insistence that decisions to limit treatment be made by patients or, in some circumstances, by intimates acting on their behalf, I have argued that decisions are, in fact, as often (or more often) made by physicians. Unable to evaluate the course of a disease or the possibility of treatment on their own, patients and their families rely on the technical judgment of physicians. But the judgment of physicians in these matters is not simply technical. It is also shaped by their own interests and by adaptations to the stresses of medical practice, as well as by apparently high-minded concerns that are at best ambiguously patient centered. Whether physicians report a patient as "terminal" or the possibility of recovery "realistic" does involve technical judgment, but technical judgment shaped by the distinctive values of their occupation.

Even more, we might argue that physicians have turned the imperatives of formal consent, whether to the initiation of new procedures or to the discontinuation of old ones, to their own purposes. Born of and sustained by a doctor-patient relationship with neither intimacy nor a great deal of trust, formal procedures may become a means by which physicians withdraw yet further from intense involvement with their patients. Protestations of patient autonomy in this context become little more than an excuse for disengagement.

Neither does the situation look very different if we go beyond informed consent or termination of treatment to questions of allocation of resources. While limited resources, whether in intensive care or elsewhere, have certainly weakened the position of physicians more generally, they may have actually strengthened the position of physicians in relation to patients. By encouraging a utilitarian ethic, limited resources undermine physicians' commitments to individual patients, allowing at least some physicians to assume a position in which they adjudicate among competing claims. The patient's position is correspondingly weakened.

In all these respects, if the intention of medical ethics as a social movement has been to empower patients, it has not succeeded. Yet simply to dismiss medical ethics as out of touch with the reality of medical practice would also be a mistake.

Medicine's Two Cultures

Much of American sociology, as Herve Varenne has observed, has been preoccupied with the "discovery of the real behind the ideal, an orientation justified by the need to ensure that political rhetoric not be mere lip service and be translated into objectively measurable reality." [1] My account of medical ethics in practice has surely shared in this preoccupation. Much of my criticism of physicians, explicit and implied, has been for their failure to live up to their own expressed ideals. With this, however, I do not mean to accuse physicians of hypocrisy—an accusation that not only would do an injustice to the deep convictions of many practitioners but also would do little to help clarify the complexities of contemporary medicine. As Varenne has also observed, ideals themselves may be real, even if they are not always translated into action.

Medical ethics has become part of the culture of medicine, particularly in the form of what I have called a culture of rights. But the culture of rights is not the only culture of medicine. There is also what might be thought of as a culture of the ward. The culture of the ward emerges much more directly than the culture of rights out of the long and insular training of medical school, internship, and residency—aspects of which I discussed in chapter 4—as well as from the everyday experience of medical practice. [2] National in

1. Herve Varenne, *Americans Together* (New York: Teachers College Press, 1977), p. 208.
2. Put a little more precisely, the culture of the ward is better understood as a subculture in the sense that it depends on "face-to-face interaction in the generation and activation of cultural elements" and then diffuses through a series of social connections "resulting in the construction

character but allowing for local variations, it is passed on from older physicians to younger ones, elaborated in jokes and stories, embedded in the special use of terms like "torture" or "terminal" and in distinctions like that between "withholding" and "withdrawing." The culture of the ward is widely shared among physicians and, to some degree, nurses. But unlike the culture of rights, lay persons are rarely participants in it.

At the core of the culture of rights, as it is written about and taught, is a distinctive emphasis on autonomy. In contrast, the culture of the ward gives far more attention to substantive (rather than procedural) matters and to technical rather than ethical considerations. Where the culture of rights allows only for patient-centered considerations, the culture of the ward allows for the stresses and strains of medical personnel and celebrates the obligations of health personnel to each other as well as to patients. But the difference between the culture of rights and the culture of the ward is not simply a matter of different values. The two cultures are also, as it were, two sets of tools that physicians use to think about different aspects of the same difficult questions.[3] In particular, the culture of rights, based on the abstract moral dicta of medical ethics, provides a set of tools for thinking about general principles. In contrast, the ward culture provides a set of tools forged in the everyday practice of medicine, appropriate for thinking about particular cases.

For many physicians, the tensions between the culture of rights and the culture of the ward are troubling. A few, struck by the incongruities between the principles of ethics and the orientations that emerge from their everyday practice, may even reject one or the other altogether—usually the culture of rights. One Outerboro attending, for example, held out practice as a far better guide than abstract speculation:

I generally do not read the medical philosophical things because I think most of them are garbage. . . . My major complaint on this is that we have people who are writing very interesting and educated sounding expositions on philosophical aspects of medical care and . . . very rarely are these people actually involved in the day-to-day practice of medicine.

Similarly, a Countryside resident who had made a special effort to take an

of a common universe of discourse throughout the social network." Gary Alan Fine and Sherryl Kleinman, "Subculture: An Interactionist Analysis," *American Journal of Sociology* 85 (1979): 1–20. See also Howard Becker, Blanche Geer, Everett Hughes, and Anselm Strauss, *Boys in White: Student Culture in Medical School* (Chicago: University of Chicago Press, 1961).

3. For the view of culture that I am drawing on here, see Ann Swidler, "Culture in Action: Symbols and Strategy," *American Sociological Review* 51 (1986): 273–86.

elective in medical ethics while in medical school now found the lessons of that elective of little help. After three years of rotations through wards and units, he had come to look elsewhere for guidance than to formal principles: "I can't imagine teaching ethics."

For others, though, the tensions are manageable, at least in the short run. Indeed, much of my account has consisted of an effort to show how physicians attempt to resolve the tensions between the culture of rights and the culture of the ward. Patients, they may acknowledge, have priority in matters of values, but physicians, they argue, have priority on questions of technique. Patients, they may acknowledge, have the right to set the general direction of medical care, but physicians, they argue, are better equipped to make specific decisions. In principle, they may acknowledge, families are best able to speak for incompetent patients, but in practice, they argue, specific families are not. "Torture," they may say, is pointless pain inflicted on patients, but they also use the term to express their own pain. Logicians might find such distinctions and elisions unsatisfactory. But for physicians themselves, like practitioners in any field, the standards of consistency are not so high.

It is not, then, simply that some physicians accept medical ethics and others reject it—although surely some do each. It is, rather, that most physicians accept both the culture of rights and the culture of the ward. The ritualistic qualities of Do Not Resuscitate orders, for example, draw on (and to some degree resolve the tensions between) both the culture of rights and the culture of the ward. Similarly, when a physician claims, as one of the residents at Countryside did, that "the decision is not mine—whose treatment should be withdrawn, who should be code or no-code," and then goes ahead and makes the decision anyway, it is not disingenuous. Rather, he is simply applying different tools to different problems—drawing on the culture of rights to think about general principles, drawing on the culture of the ward to think about particular cases. This is not hypocrisy, only the normal confusion that accompanies the equally fervid belief in two often incompatible positions.

Medicine without Legitimacy

If, in the short run, physicians can tolerate a fairly high level of inconsistency, the situation, in the only slightly longer run, may be quite different. In the very course of making the accommodations to medical ethics that allow them to maintain much of their discretion in the day-to-day practice of medicine, physicians may be conceding claims that are themselves the source of that discretion.

Most important, physicians may be in the process of maintaining their discretion only by conceding their authority. It has long been characteristic of American professions more generally to use technical skill as the basis for claims to moral authority. Certainly over the course of the first half of the twentieth century, medicine did so. In its ascendance, medicine used technical expertise not only to carve out an area in which physicians could act independently but also to establish grounds on which lay people would accept their jurisdiction. The triumph of medicine depended, then, not just on the efficacy of medicine's technical skills but also on a faith in science—a belief, undemonstrated and perhaps undemonstrable, that science, manifest in medicine, could solve a remarkably wide range of human problems. Today, however, science has for the most part lost its charms. And, within medicine, medical ethics has played its part in breaking our faith.

At the core of much of contemporary medical ethics is a fairly sharp distinction between matters of technique and matters of value. "The questions at stake" in contemporary medical ethics are, as Robert Veatch has written, "fundamentally philosophical or ethical. That they arise in a medical context should not lead anyone to conclude that they are the exclusive purview of the scientific expert. They are in but not of the realm of science."[4] Physicians, however, as I have shown at great length throughout this book, often deny this distinction in practice, moving more and more into the realm of technical medicine and away from the realm of ethics. But at the same, as I have also shown at length, physicians accept the distinction in principle. "I think it is possible to separate the medical and the ethical," one resident told me. Certainly, both he and his colleagues do so frequently, not only in their unrelenting fealty to principles of patients' rights but also in their insistent questions to patients and families about what they want and in their ritualized recording of patients' preferences in orders not to resuscitate—all the while reserving to themselves judgments about which drug to use or which procedure to adopt. Physicians, then, continue to make decisions for patients but with dramatically reduced claims that they have a right to do so.

In the short run, the accommodation makes good sense from the point of view of physicians. What difference does it make, after all, to concede a principle if at the same time you can treat patients you want to treat, avoid treating

4. Robert Veatch, *Death, Dying, and the Biological Revolution* (New Haven: Yale University Press, 1976), p. 18.

patients you don't want to treat, and escape the pain of confronting the futility of medical measures? In the long run, however, the accommodation is dangerous. By conceding that they have no right to make decisions in matters of ethics and values, physicians leave themselves open to counterclaims that the realm of technical judgment should be narrowed. These counterclaims come not only from without (whether from ethicists, courts, or patients themselves) but also from within, from physicians who, precisely because they do take principles seriously, are prepared to exercise a self-restraint virtually unknown to physicians even in the recent past.

This strategy is all the more dangerous to the authority of physicians because it is also one that seems to have been adopted by much of medicine's leadership. While many of these leaders are surely sympathetic to the culture of the ward, only a few have defended it publicly—perhaps because the ward culture's basis in everyday practice leaves it peculiarly unsuited to principled formulations.[5] In contrast, the culture of rights has attracted a great deal of support. In endorsing formal procedures for informed consent and termination of treatment—as they have in the hospitals they manage, the societies they run, and the reports they write—many of medicine's leaders may be attempting to forestall even greater regulation by reforming themselves from within. In accepting distinctions between ethics and medicine, between questions of value and those of technique, these leaders may be attempting to define an area of expertise that is medicine's and medicine's alone. But this is the strategy of a profession in decline, no longer attempting to extend its authority and fighting a rearguard action to defend a reduced part of its authority against the encroachments of ethicists, courts, and patients.

Only around questions of allocating resources has medicine assumed a more aggressive stance. By developing convincing measures of medical outcomes—whether for ICUs in particular or for medical interventions more generally—physicians are reasserting the significance of technical medical knowledge as a guide to public policy. As John—the director of the Countryside ICU and the most articulate proponent of this position among the physicians I studied—insisted, "Medicine should take the leadership in this. . . . The physician needs to take the leadership position." By accumulating data, John implied, echoing a strategy that at least a few physicians have assumed

5. For two important exceptions, see Franz Ingelfinger, "Arrogance," *New England Journal of Medicine* 303 (1980): 1507–11, and David Jackson and Stuart Youngner, "Patient Autonomy and Death with Dignity: Some Clinical Caveats," *New England Journal of Medicine* 301 (1979): 404–8.

at a national level, physicians can reassert their authority even in the face of attacks:

What if we say that patients with cirrhosis and pneumonia have a 20 percent recovery rate, and government wants to cut off care for cirrhosis patients? We can use the data and say, "Well, we have data on patients who are very sick and come in with a chronic disease and I know you don't want to treat alcoholic cirrhotics but here's the data. These patients have a 20 percent survival." . . . I think the standard should be appropriateness of medical care. . . . We could say it on a public policy basis from the medical societies.

Such dreams of the philosopher doctor notwithstanding, even this strategy has its limits. In the first instance, the development of outcome measures as a guide to decisions, with its suggestion of gatekeepers operating at a national level as well as at the level of the hospital, implies a stratification of the profession alien to medical traditions. As I suggested in the previous chapter, it is likely to meet with fierce resistance from individual practitioners insistent on defending their own prerogatives in making decisions for their own patients. In the second instance, it is a strategy limited to issues bearing on the allocation of resources. Although such issues are likely to grow in importance over the coming years, there are no signs of an equivalent strategy by which physicians could reassert the significance of medical expertise in matters bearing more directly on the choices individual patients have been given the mandate to make. And, most important, the development of outcome measures, even with its appearance of physicians reasserting their preeminence, implies an acceptance of medicine's new limits. It is a strategy physicians turn to only as they acknowledge that medicine will not command the seemingly unbounded resources it once enjoyed. This too, then, is a strategy of the rear guard.

The future is both unknown and unknowable. And those who risk projecting the present into the future do so with the certainty only of embarrassment as the unforeseen becomes real. If, for example, the costs of medical care continue to grow, creating additional strains on an already fragile economy, the balance of authority may well switch back toward physicians, acting not as advocates for individual patients but as gatekeepers for increasingly scarce resources. Increased financial stringency may well, then, generate pressures for what the ethicist Paul Ramsey has called a "medical indications policy"—a policy that within the bounds of permissible action "the physician should do what is medically indicated," based on criteria of the ability to extend life and reduce disability. This policy would, in effect, turn judgment back to technical determinations of the sort that physicians are uniquely competent to make.[6] But this is only one possible scenario and not in my judgment the likeliest.

Whatever else, the tensions between patient autonomy and medical discretion are unlikely to disappear. Although more (and better) laws, court decisions, and hospital policies may well remove questions of informed consent and termination of treatment from their now prominent position in public discourse, they are unlikely to resolve the underlying tension. That tension is rooted deep in the structure of contemporary medicine, in a structure that produces encounters between physicians and patients whose interests diverge and who neither know nor trust each other.

Within this are clues to the future of medicine as a profession. That future will not, of course, depend solely or even primarily on the issues that have animated medical ethics. The rise of medical ethics is, itself, as much a symptom as a cause of medicine's waning authority. Equally important, if not more so, are developments in the financial regulation of medicine, transformations in the structure of medical practice, the ability of medical schools to continue to attract the excellent students that have characterized their recent past, the impact of AIDS, the impact of new medical technologies, and much more. Yet medical ethics will play its part. Insofar as the tension between patient autonomy and medical discretion helps shape medicine's future, there is little place for apocalyptic visions of precipitous decline.[7] The technical knowledge of physicians equips them with too powerful a resource to allow them to become mere mechanics of the body. Not only will physicians continue to offer their skills, but in offering those skills they will continue to shape the choices of the patients who are their putative masters. But neither will medicine be what it once was. If physicians continue to shape the choices of their patients, they will do so more or less covertly. If nothing else, the rise of medical ethics seems to have put to rest the type of medical arrogance that insisted not only on making decisions but on the right to make those decisions. The vision of the doctor as philosopher or the doctor as priest may not have vanished entirely, but it has, at the very least, grown blurry.

6. Paul Ramsey, *Ethics at the Edge of Life* (New Haven: Yale University Press, 1978); Thomas M. Garrett, Harold W. Baillie, and Rosellen M. Garrett, *Health Care Ethics* (Englewood Cliffs, NJ: Prentice Hall, 1989), p. 59.

7. See, for example, John B. McKinley and Joan Arches, "Towards the Proletarianization of Physicians," *International Journal of Health Services* 15 (1985): 161–95. For more temperate analyses, see Eliot Freidson, "The Reorganization of the Medical Profession," *Medical Care Review* 42 (1985): 11–35, and Charles Derber, "Sponsorship and the Control of Physicians," *Theory and Society* 12 (1983): 561–601.

In contrast, the future of medical ethics seems bright. With all of its failings, most importantly its frequent failure to connect with the realities of medical practice, medical ethics has nonetheless accomplished a great deal. While only a minority of patients are likely ever to take advantage of the rights the medical ethics movement has helped win for them, those who wish to are now better able to do so. While many physicians continue to rail against the presence of ethicists in their schools and hospitals and against the interventions of courts and lawmakers, most have embraced at least some of the perspectives characteristic of the movement. They have done so not because of formal or specific rules of the sort sometimes favored by ethicists and lawmakers. Rather, they have done so because ethicists and lawmakers, along with hospital administrators and many physicians themselves, have insistently placed matters of ethics on the agenda of medical training and medical practice. The questions, as it were, have mattered more than the answers, and the movement has triumphed in spirit if not always in substance.

None of this is to guarantee that medical ethics will continue to play the prominent part in medicine that it has in recent decades. In the past, other disciplines have appeared in medical schools with the promise of providing special insights unavailable from the study of physiology or pharmacology alone—only to fall by the wayside, eliminated from the medical school curriculum and the medical vision in favor of some other, more recent trend. Medical ethics may be no more than a successor to the behavioral sciences or psychology as medicine's brief bow to the world beyond its boundaries, fated eventually like its predecessors to be confined to the margins of medical consciousness. But even this seems unlikely. For better or for worse—or for both—medical ethics has entered the discourse of medical practice.

Appendix: On Method

The research reported in this book represents the results of my third extended effort as a field-worker.[1] By current standards in sociology, this constitutes a great deal of experience.[2] I am not, however, very comfortable with an attempt to lay out any general principles about fieldwork as a method. The reason is simple. Fieldwork is not a method. Rather, fieldwork, at least as the

1. For reports of my earlier research, see Robert Zussman, *Mechanics of the Middle Class* (Berkeley: University of California Press, 1985), and chapter 7 of David Rothman and Sheila Rothman, *The Willowbrook Wars* (New York: Harper & Row, 1984). The sociological study of medicine has attracted more than its share of excellent fieldwork. See, for example, Howard Becker, Blanche Geer, Everett Hughes, and Anselm Strauss, *Boys in White: Student Culture in Medical School* (Chicago: University of Chicago Press, 1961); Charles Bosk, *Forgive and Remember: Managing Medical Failure* (Chicago: University of Chicago Press, 1979); Rose Coser, *Life in the Ward* (East Lansing: Michigan State University Press, 1962); Renee Fox, *Experiment Perilous* (Glencoe, IL: Free Press, 1959); Renee Fox and Judith Swazey, *The Courage to Fail*, 2d ed. (Chicago: University of Chicago Press, 1978); Eliot Freidson, *Doctoring Together: A Study of Professional Social Control* (Chicago: University of Chicago Press, 1975); Barney Glaser and Anselm Strauss, *Awareness of Dying* (Chicago: Aldine, 1965); Jeanne Harley Guilleman and Lynda Lytle Holmstrom, *Mixed Blessings: Intensive Care for Newborns* (New York: Oxford University Press, 1986); Charles W. Lidz and Alan Meisel with Janice L. Holden, John H. Marx, and Mark Munetz, "Informed Consent and the Structure of Medical Care," in President's Commission for the Study of Ethical Problems in Medicine and Biomedical and Behavioral Research, *Making Health Care Decisions*, vol. 2: *Appendices, Empirical Studies of Informed Consent* (Washington, DC: Government Printing Office, 1982), pp. 317–410; Robert Merton, George Reader, and Patricia Kendall, eds., *The Student Physician* (Cambridge, MA: Harvard University Press, 1957); Marcia Millman, *The Unkindest Cut* (New York: Morrow, 1977); Terry Mizrahi, *Getting Rid of Patients* (New Brunswick, NJ: Rutgers University Press, 1986); Diana Scully, *Men Who Control Women's Health: The Miseducation of Obstetricians and Gynecologists* (Boston: Houghton Mifflin, 1980); Anselm Strauss, Shizuko Fagerhaugh, Barbara Suczek, and Carolyn Wiener, *Social Organization of Medical Work* (Chicago: University of Chicago Press, 1985).

2. Although the claim would be difficult to document, it is my impression that (with a good number of notable exceptions) an unusually high proportion of sociologists who have produced superb first books based on fieldwork have then either failed to produce second books, taken a very long time to do so, or turned to different methods. I suspect that most of us, myself very much included, simply find fieldwork too exhausting, too time consuming (especially if undertaken in conjunction with a full-time teaching position), and too inefficient to justify the effort.

term is conventionally used, refers to virtually any method of data collection in which the researcher observes the subjects of his or her research in more or less natural settings. Data collected by a field-worker may be easily quantifiable or it may defy quantification. It may be highly idiosyncratic or easily replicated. It may be exploratory or it may be definitive (at least as definitive as any sociological research ever is). At the same time, many of the issues that animate accounts of fieldwork—questions of observer bias or about the ability to generalize—are appropriate to virtually all kinds of sociological research. In my view, then, it is not possible to provide a general defense of fieldwork, at least not outside a general treatise on method. Neither, though, is it necessary. Although some would make a cult of fieldwork and others would reject it out of hand, my view is that it is simply one method among many of collecting data.

If fieldwork in general neither needs nor lends itself to justification, I am nonetheless under some obligation to explain my own procedures. As in any research, I am obliged to explain how I know what I claim to know. What follows, then, is an account of what I did, how I did it, why I did it, and what I think it all adds up to. If other field-workers find this account helpful in thinking about their own research, so much the better. But that is not my primary aim. Rather, my aim is only to explain myself.

What I Did

This book began, in effect, with my appointment in 1983 as an assistant professor of social medicine at the then newly formed Center for the Study of Society and Medicine in the Department of Medicine at Columbia University. Although the center's mandate was loose and (appropriately) ill defined, one matter was clear. We were expected to teach and conduct research in the general area of medical ethics. There was nothing peculiar in this mandate. Over the last decade many other medical schools have devised similar centers with similar mandates. What was peculiar, however, was the relationship between this mandate and the training of the center's staff. The director of the center was (and is) David Rothman, a historian. The other assistant professor, besides myself, was Sherry Brandt-Rauf, a lawyer with graduate training in sociology. None of us, with the only partial exception of Brandt-Rauf, had a well-defined prior interest in medicine. Even more clearly, none of us was inclined to the type of normative thought that characterizes most academic work in medical ethics. Given our backgrounds, the center quickly took on a distinctive intellectual style. We would not "do ethics," at least in the way ethicists and philosophers do ethics. Rather, we would study ethics as an empirical phenomenon, as part of the changing world of medicine (and a changing world the center was itself a part of).

From the beginning of his appointment as director of the center, Rothman had settled on the habit of attending morning rounds on the medical service of Columbia-Presbyterian Hospital (the primary affiliate of the Columbia medical school) as a way of acquainting himself with medical practice. When Brandt-Rauf and I joined the center a few months later, we took up Rothman's practice. A few months later, at Rothman's suggestion, I began rounding in the Intensive Care Unit. Although, for reasons of confidentiality, I have not included the results of my first ventures into the ICU at my home institution, the time I spent there was critical in forming the ideas and insights that guided my later research at Outerboro and Countryside.

I began my research at Outerboro in earnest in September of 1985. I had negotiated entrée to the unit through the director of the medical service and Dennis, the unit director. Dennis had been unenthusiastic about the project, concerned (reasonably) that my presence might interfere with the central clinical tasks of the unit. He agreed to my presence only after the director of the medical service and the hospital's president intervened. Their intervention, I suspect, was prompted not only by a desire to maintain good relations with the nearby Columbia medical school but also by a commitment, characteristic of American teaching hospitals more generally, to research.

Once I had gained entrée, I began rounding in nineteen-day stretches (from a Monday through the third Friday). I repeated this procedure six times at Outerboro over two years. The patients admitted to or discharged from the unit on days I was rounding make up my sample of 233 admissions and 237 discharges. Rounds, I should note, are a remarkable institution, the sort of thing sociologists would want to invent for research if physicians had not already invented them for their own purposes. Certainly there are ceremonial elements in rounds. Standing at the patient's bedside, speaking without looking at their notes, housestaff perform for attendings. Attendings perform for housestaff. And, to some extent (although less so in the ICU than elsewhere), housestaff and attendings perform for patients, enacting, as it were, the seriousness of their efforts. Rounds do not consist of "backstage" behavior. Coarse language, black humor, and bitter complaints, occasional during rounds, are all more frequent during informal conversations and (for the housestaff) in the absence of attendings. But these qualifications notwithstanding, rounds provide access to medical thinking of a sort available nowhere else. While rounds are not public in the sense that anyone may attend, they are public in the sense that usually tacit thought processes are made explicit. Called on to propose or defend a course of action, an intern or resident has to explain his or her logic. So, too, must an attending, whether proposing an alternative course of action, suggesting an additional consideration, or simply teaching. Rounds, then, provide an opportunity to hear doctors, in effect, think out loud.

While on rounds, I took notes selectively. In particular, I did not make an effort to record a great deal of discussions that were primarily technical, for example, of the effectiveness of one drug rather than another, of different methods of mechanical ventilation, or of different diagnostic techniques. Much of these discussions I simply did not understand; much, I was not interested in. I did, however, record every mention of families or friends, every mention of cost, every discussion of getting the patient's (or family's) consent, and every discussion of limiting potentially life-prolonging treatment. In taking notes, I made every effort to record discussions in a form as close to word for word as I could.

I made no effort to record summaries of cases or discussions and no effort to record my own interpretations. In earlier research (on technical workers in industry), I had made such efforts and found that I knew a great deal. But I often found myself unable to reproduce the process by which I had come to know what I believed I knew in a way that would convince anyone else. As a result, in the ICU I concentrated my efforts exclusively on collecting data—words and actions—that could stand on their own apart from my interpretation of them. To be sure, no data stand entirely on their own apart from the interpretive scheme, theoretical and common sense, that the researcher brings to them. But some data come closer. My understanding of an event is not subject to reinterpretation (except insofar as I am the object of research); what someone said or wrote is. While I am by no means convinced that what someone wrote or said explicitly is ultimately more valid— "truer"—than what I have come to understand from what is implicit, it is certainly more usable data and, at least in the rhetoric of the social sciences, more convincing.

For the most part my note taking caused little comment. Housestaff themselves frequently take notes during rounds, primarily on what they have to do after rounds. As a result, my note taking, although much more extensive than that of the housestaff, probably did not seem entirely out of place. Occasionally, an intern or resident peeked over my shoulder to see what I was writing. A few asked me directly what I was writing. On all such occasions, I simply showed my notes to whoever was curious. Although my handwriting is not easy to read, no one ever asked me to decipher it. I suspect that my willing-ness to reveal my notes was sufficient to allay any fears. In some cases, I added a brief explanation. If anyone had been curious enough to ask, I would have provided a longer explanation. No one was.

I was unobtrusive during rounds in other respects, as well. Dennis had made it clear that, while he had agreed to my attending rounds, he expected me not to participate. This expectation I met, not only because it was a con-dition of my attendance but also because it made good sense as a research strategy. I wanted to see medicine as it is practiced, not as it is practiced in the presence of someone perceived as an ethicist.[3] Although I did frequently ask one of the housestaff or, less frequently, one of the attendings to explain something that had just been said, I did so in asides, in private conversations, usually while walking from one bed to another. I never addressed comments or questions to the rounding physicians as a group. Occasionally during rounds, the Outerboro attendings did address comments to me about topics they thought might be of special interest. But these comments were few and far between. I have neither record nor memory that any of the housestaff or nurses ever addressed remarks to me during rounds.

During rounds I wore a tie but no jacket, a fashion adopted by some of the male housestaff and a few of the attendings. (Other modes of dress in-cluded, in various combination, a white jacket, no tie, and surgical scrubs.) In her 1962 study *Life in the Ward*, Rose Coser reported that, on the advice of nurses, she wore a white coat, which "served to identify me as one of the professional personnel."[4] Although Coser's procedure made good sense in the context of the 1950s (when she conducted her research), it would have been hard to justify in the 1980s. It would seem a type of deception entirely out of the spirit of notions of informed consent and patients' rights. By dressing in the manner of housestaff without wearing a white coat, I was able to make myself unobtrusive without claiming to be something I was not. In this minor sense, my research procedures reflected the very phenomenon—the rise of medical ethics—I had set out to study.

After rounds at Outerboro, I usually retreated to the doctors' conference room, reviewing charts while the attendings and housestaff wrote their own notes. Late in the afternoon or in the early evening, as my other responsibil-ities permitted, I sometimes returned to the unit to continue chart reviews.

3. For an experiment along these lines, see Bernard Lo and Steven A. Schroeder, "Fre-quency of Ethical Dilemmas in a Medical Inpatient Service," *Archives of Internla Medicine* 141 (1981): 1062–64.
4. Coser, *Life in the Ward*, p. xxi.

Reviewing charts served four purposes. First, it provided background that helped me understand cases that had been discussed on rounds. Second, as discussed in chapter 12, charts are an important part of medical discourse, supplementary to but distinct from discussions on rounds or more private conversations. Third, along with data collected later from the two hospitals' computerized records, charts are my primary source of basic demographic information about the units' patients and about hospital admissions and discharges. Fourth (and not least), reviewing charts gave me a legitimate reason for spending more time in the units, an opportunity I used to engage housestaff, attendings, and nurses in more casual conversation than was possible at other times.

I have no way of knowing the housestaff's first impressions of me. I suspect they considered me a slight curiosity. If I had been studying authority relations between attendings and housestaff, coming in under the aegis of the unit's director might have caused some concern.[5] But I was introduced and introduced myself as someone studying ethics, which in fact I was. In any event, the housestaff became quite accustomed to me. I had originally settled on the pattern of rounding for nineteen consecutive days to establish continuity. (If I missed one day, not only did I miss what happened on the day I was out but I had more difficulty following what happened the day I returned.) But I soon discovered that the pattern had another advantage as well. It convinced the housestaff and the nurses that I was serious. On one Sunday at Countryside, early on in my research, one of the residents showed surprise at seeing me in the unit: "You spend almost as much time here as we do." From a harried resident, it was a high compliment. It was also an advantage that my research at Outerboro stretched over two years. By the end, I had simply become a familiar part of the unit. "I think you were there long enough that we got used to you," one Outerboro resident told me. "Now, this year's senior residents are more used to having you there. . . . You were sort of always there so it didn't bother us."

I cannot claim that I liked all of the housestaff. Some, I suspect, did not like me. Most, however, I got along with well and those good relations stood me in good stead. Contemporary medicine is complicated. As a sociologist without any formal training in medicine, as someone who had not even taken a course in biology since high school, I often found myself unable to follow many cases. (The various medical texts, nursing texts, and guides for housestaff that I read assiduously provided only episodic help.) My response was

5. See Bosk, *Forgive and Remember.*

to ask questions, occasionally of attendings, very occasionally of nurses, most often of housestaff. It was my good fortune that they usually answered patiently and informatively, explaining not only the relevant technical issues but also the sometimes coded language in which they discussed limiting treatment and other issues bearing directly on matters of ethics. I could not have conducted the research without their help.

Only after I had already "rotated" through the unit twice did I begin interviewing. I began with the housestaff because I knew them best and eventually completed twenty interviews with residents I had observed rotating through the unit. Although I entered the interview with a schedule, the interviews were open-ended and I often departed from the schedule. Moreover, I included in each interview a number of questions about particular cases I knew the resident had been involved with. Because I knew the residents, I was also able to take certain liberties during the interviews. In particular, I occasionally argued. Although this is not a technique that I would recommend in most situations, it worked well with the Outerboro residents—not only because we already knew each other but also because they are, as a group, unusually self-confident and assertive. By arguing (albeit good-naturedly), I was able to force them to make their points more explicit and to refine distinctions. I also conducted formal interviews with four physicians who attended in the unit and a series of intensive interviews with one intern I had come to know well.

I began interviewing nurses soon after I began interviewing the housestaff. Although I had spent considerable time talking to some of the nurses informally, I had not observed the nurses as intensively as I had observed the housestaff. Although the nurses as a group do have occasional meetings (a few of which I attended), they are more for the purposes of discussing general unit nursing policy (ranging from new protocols for administering drugs to vacation time) than for the discussion of particular cases. There is no equivalent in ICU nursing to the physicians' teaching rounds. As a result, I did not know most of the nurses as well as I knew the physicians. I had, however, by the time I began my interviews, been around the unit long enough so that most of the nurses knew who I was and, at least vaguely, what I was doing. Like the interviews with housestaff, the interviews with nurses were open-ended. In all, I completed twenty interviews with Outerboro nurses.

I had originally hoped to complete my research at Outerboro by interviewing both patients and their families. But both the unit director and the chief of medical services were uncomfortable with my interviewing families.

Both did eventually agree to my conducting such interviews but only after I had myself proposed fairly restrictive conditions. In the case of patients who died in the hospital, for example, I agreed to postpone any interviews with family until a minimum of six months after the death and then approach the family initially by mail. In the end, these conditions proved too cumbersome and I conducted no interviews with families of Outerboro patients. I was, however (with the assistance of Jonathan Sharpe, then a medical student at Columbia), able to interview twenty patients. Although I have called on these interviews at various points in this book, particularly in part I, they were, in my judgment, the least successful part of the research. Although I limited my interviews to patients who had apparently been awake and alert during their ICU stay, even many of these could not remember the unit clearly. As a result, many of the patients simply had very little to say.

When I completed my research at Outerboro in August of 1987 and prepared to move to a new position in the Department of Sociology at SUNY-Stony Brook, I thought I was finished with fieldwork. Although I would have liked to add a second research site, I suspected that my teaching responsibilities at Stony Brook would keep me from doing so. I was prepared to write up what I had already done and leave matters at that. But in December of 1987 I received a call from the National Center for Health Services Research informing me that I had been awarded a grant that I had first applied for years earlier. That grant, along with additional funding from the Picker Foundation and Stony Brook's generous leave policy, allowed me to take a year off from teaching and conduct my research at Countryside.

Where my entrée to Outerboro had been preceded by protracted negotiations, my entrée to Countryside was remarkably simple. A friend at a Massachusetts university had given me the name of the Countryside unit's director. I wrote John a brief letter explaining my research, I called a few days later, and we had lunch together a few days after that. To my astonishment, John agreed immediately to my studying his unit. Although I did have to go through various other approvals in the hospital, none presented any difficulty. Getting into the Countryside unit proved to be even simpler than getting into the Outerboro unit had proved difficult.

Once inside Countryside, I followed roughly the same research procedures I had established at Outerboro but with a few key differences. I did not think, and do not think now, that my research at the two hospitals required exact symmetry. In some instances, the differences in my research procedures were a response to genuinely different conditions at Countryside. In others, they were a response to my own research needs. Most important, I had already learned a great deal at Outerboro that I did not have to relearn at Countryside.

Although I maintained my practice of rounding in the unit for nineteen-day stretches, I limited my number of "rotations" to three. Over fifty-seven days, I observed 117 admissions and 117 discharges, a smaller sample than I had at Outerboro but sufficient to draw comparisons. Although I spent fewer days at Countryside than at Outerboro, the days I spent there were longer. Because Countryside had afternoon as well as morning rounds (and because I was on leave from teaching), I usually spent the entire day in the unit, often until early evening. (At Countryside, as at Outerboro, I also made it a point to make occasional late-night visits and, once in each unit, to stay the entire night with the housestaff.)

The most important difference between Countryside and Outerboro may well have been that John, the unit director, and Ken, the unit medical director, not only were much friendlier toward me and more interested in my research than all but one of the Outerboro attendings but also, as full-time intensivists, spent considerably more time in the unit than any of the Outerboro attendings. To be sure, a few of the Outerboro attendings occasionally treated me as a confidant in the sense that they would say things to me they would not say to the housestaff. But John and Ken treated me, at times, as a colleague. Both took an active interest in my research and took me aside frequently to explain decisions they had made and the reasoning behind them. Both were willing to listen to and—even better—argue with my interpretations of events. Ken and I, for example, discussed collaborating on an article. Although we did not follow up on the project, the mere fact that we considered it suggests something of the tone of the relationship. Moreover, both Ken and John not only addressed comments to me during rounds but, on a few occasions, solicited my opinion on matters bearing explicitly on ethics. (I invariably said that I didn't know what to do, which was equally invariably the case.)

John's and Ken's sympathy for my project made it possible for me to conduct family interviews of the sort that I had not been able to conduct at Outerboro. John, in particular, made it a point to introduce me to families after asking if they would be willing to talk to me. Ken and a number of housestaff also provided introductions. As a result, I was able to complete fourteen interviews with family or friends of unit patients.

While the Countryside family interviews added an element that had been missing in my research at Outerboro, I interviewed fewer patients (a half dozen) and fewer housestaff (also a half dozen). I did not pursue patient interviews aggressively because I had not found them useful at Outerboro and saw no reason why either the quality of the interviews or the character of the patients would be different at Countryside. In the case of housestaff, the number available for interviews was limited by the number of housestaff I observed—a number significantly lower than at Outerboro because of the shorter time I spent in the unit—the longer time of housestaff rotations (a month rather than two weeks), and the smaller number of housestaff in the unit at any one time (three interns rather than four, one resident rather than three). If I had seen indications that the Countryside housestaff differed from the Outerboro housestaff in any systematic way, if they had demonstrated significantly different orientations, attitudes, or insights, I might have pursued additional interviews. But I saw few indications of such differences.

In the case of nurses, I did see significant differences between Countryside and Outerboro, some of which I discussed in chapter 5. As a result—especially since interviews were my primary source of data about nursing—I did interview as many nurses at Outerboro (twenty) as I had at Countryside.

One final note on data collection: both Outerboro and Countryside, like formal organizations everywhere, generate a great number of written documents, in the form of memos, policy statements, and guides for staff and patients. Although I cannot claim to have reviewed these materials systematically, I did ask to see those I knew of and thought would be relevant to my purposes. Although this material, which I have cited at various points throughout the text, would not stand easily on its own, it constitutes a useful supplement to other sources of data.

Although a great deal has been written about the collection of data in the field, surprisingly little has been written about the analysis of that data. In large part, I suspect, this is because there are few satisfactory techniques. Data that could be quantified posed no special problems. Data that could not be quantified—my notes from rounds and most interview material—did. I was fortunate to have sufficient funding to have all of my interviews transcribed on a personal computer. (Or, more accurately, I had transcribed all interviews that were audible on the mediocre tape recorder that, in an instance of unusually bad judgment, I used.) I typed my field notes myself.[6]

---

6. By the time I arrived at Countryside I had acquired a laptop. I thought I would use the laptop to type up my notes immediately after rounds and to record material from charts at bedside—thus skipping the stage of copying chart material into a notebook before entering it into the computer. I soon discovered, however, that, as soon as I sat down at bedside with the laptop, I wound up spending more time discussing computers than I did reviewing charts. Although I continued to use the laptop, I did so discreetly, usually in a corner of the doctor's conference

Having entered interviews and my notes onto a computer, I then regrouped the material around substantive themes, first at the level of a chapter, then at the level of a chapter subheading. (Perhaps needless to say, I also did a great deal of shuffling among categories.) Moreover, before writing any particular sections I supplemented my first effort at coding with word searches for specific terms or phrases relevant to it. For example, for a page or two that I wrote on doctors' views of nurses, I was able, in a matter of a half hour or so, to generate some forty pages of transcripts by searching through the physician interviews for any mention of nurses. Similarly, before writing the chapter on the effects of law on ICU practice, I did word searches for "law," "legal," and "courts." I do not, however, want to overemphasize the value of computerized methods of analyzing text. In the end, two tools are more important than any others. One is memory. The other is reading through the texts over and over and over. Computers, sadly, are no substitute for either.

What It Means

But what does it all mean? I did not set out to complete an ethnography of intensive care, to capture the total life of the unit. I was not interested, for example, in the large number of ancillary personnel—technicians, cleaning people, ward clerks, among others—who work in the unit but are not involved in any meaningful way in making medical decisions. Neither was I interested in the training of physicians and nurses or the relationships among health personnel except as such issues formed the context for my primary interests. Rather, I approached Outerboro and Countryside as strategic research sites which would allow me to answer a series of more specific questions. In particular, I was interested in studying two intensive care units as a way of learning something about the relationship between medical ethics and the practice of medicine. How successful my strategy was for these purposes depends on the answer to one question: How generalizable are my findings?

The question of generalization is itself composed of a number of different questions, each appropriate to a different level of research. On one level, I have various samples of individuals—of doctors, nurses, patients, families, cases. At another level, I have a sample of only two organizations. At the first level, the appropriate question is how well my various samples represent the relevant populations of people or events within each organization. At the sec-

---

room and among people who were used to seeing both me and my then still novel piece of equipment.

ond level, the appropriate question is both how well the two units represent intensive care more generally and how well intensive care represents American medicine more generally.

Only in the instances of my admission and discharge samples along with the analysis of the relationship between empty beds and admissions (in which the unit of analysis is the day) introduced in chapter 14 would I claim that any of my findings are generalizable in a statistical sense. And even in these instances I must acknowledge that I can generalize only to Outerboro and Countryside, not beyond.

I would not claim that my "samples" of either doctors, nurses, patients, or patients' families are representative even of the relevant populations at the two units. Although only one doctor (an Outerboro resident) and no nurses refused my request for an interview, I did not approach either doctors or nurses systematically with requests for interviews. In particular, I was much likelier to approach those nurses whom I had already met and who had shown some interest in my research than those I had not met and who had not shown interest. Similarly among patients and families, I was probably somewhat more likely to interview those without a private physician than those with one, if only because the process of getting permission to approach the patient or family member (part of the research protocol at both hospitals) was administratively simpler when the primary physician was a member of the housestaff routinely in the hospital rather than an often difficult to find private. Moreover, the numbers in each group are small. As a result, I avoided, entirely self-consciously, quantifying interviews. To be sure, I have occasionally made quasi-quantitative claims from the interviews—using phrases like "most," "more," "a few," or, for that matter, "occasionally." But such phrases seem to me preferable to a false precision of dubious significance. (The difference, for example, between 50 percent and 65 percent of twenty interviews is only three cases.)

Statistical generalization is not, however, the only form of generalization. First, my interviews allow me to say something about the *range* of responses among doctors, nurses, patients, and families. Given that I cannot easily move from statistical generalization about these populations at each hospital to generalizations about those populations beyond the two hospitals, specification of a range seems all that is reasonable in any event.

Second and, in my view, more important, my interviews allow me to say something about the logic of response. Doctors and nurses do not just come to decisions; they come to considered decisions, decisions based on more or less thoroughly considered and more or less explicit principles. While going on rounds allowed me to observe the range of contingencies (social and medical) that confront physicians and nurses and following cases allowed me to see the range of responses to those contingencies, interviews allowed me to probe the logic underlying those responses.

There are (undoubtedly among many others) two very different types of interviewing. One is sample interviewing. The other is informant interviewing. In sample interviewing, each interview is as important as every other interview. The point is to count responses and to compare distributions among subpopulations distinguished by one or another critical variable. Informant interviewing is different. Some interviews are more important than others because the respondent knows more, has better insight, or is more willing to share what he or she knows with the interviewer. In the case of my physician and nurse interviews, some interviews were more valuable than others because the respondent was better able to articulate the principles underlying decisions. Informant interviewing is especially useful when addressed to collective processes or events. The respondent is invited, as it were, to collaborate on the analysis of what happened. Here the point is not to count responses but to assemble explanations, usually from multiple perspectives.

In my use of interview materials, there is a tension between the style of sample interviewing and the style of informant interviewing. In my use of patient and family interviews I have tended to resolve that tension in favor of treating them as a sample. To be sure, there are a few instances—most notably in my discussion of Kelly Connors—in which I have been able to join patients' or families' discussions of their own cases to physicians' handling of those cases. But patients' and families' responses to the ICU are shaped by much that was extraneous to my research, by their backgrounds, by their experiences of illness, and by much else. Undoubtedly, there are collective elements in patients' and families' responses to the ICU but there is not, at least not in the ICU, a collectivity of patients themselves. Their experience of the ICU is primarily as individuals or individual families.

Doctors and nurses are different. They talk to each other, influence each other, and come to decisions in groups. Implicit in much of what I have argued is an assumption that each unit has a collective style of decision making, albeit with frequent variations. As a result (especially in part 2), I have treated the interviews of nurses, even more of housestaff, and almost entirely of attendings, as informant interviews rather than sample interviews. In this sense, each interview becomes part of an effort to make sense of a single style of decision making rather than an independent case. And insofar as there are collective styles of decision making, I do not have so many cases of nurses, so many cases of housestaff, so many cases of attendings. I have only two cases—Outerboro and Countryside—of which the nurses, housestaff, and attendings are part.

The significance of my arguments (in the substantive, not the statistical, sense) rests, then, on the representativeness of the Outerboro and Country-side ICUs. Outerboro and Countryside are not, to be sure, typical hospitals. Both Outerboro and Countryside are teaching hospitals and, as such, represent only a minority of American hospitals. Both are large, in the top 10 percent of all American hospitals as measured by number of beds. Neither are ICUs typical of hospitals. As I took pains to argue in chapter 2, they are denser in technology and personnel; their beds are more in demand; and questions about the limits of medical efforts at the end of life are more pressing. Yet it is precisely the atypicality of the hospitals and of ICUs within hospitals that makes them interesting.

Innovation in medicine, in matters of policy as well as technique, flows from larger hospitals to smaller ones, from teaching hospitals to nonteaching hospitals. As a result, if Outerboro and Countryside do not represent current practices at all hospitals, they are more likely to represent what those practices will become. A similar consideration applies to the relationship between ICUs and hospitals. Because of the density of technology, because of the collective character of decision making, because of the insistent intrusion of questions about triage and the limitation of treatment, the doctors and nurses who work in ICUs are more likely to have thought through issues that only marginally confront doctors and nurses who work elsewhere. Insofar as there is a logic to decision making, general not just to individual physicians and nurses or even to particular units but to medicine as a whole, the ICU will be among the best places to see it articulated.

I do not, of course, mean to imply that there is a single logic common to all of medicine, waiting to be uncovered. There is not. Certainly, there are significant variations, as is very much in evidence in the contrasts I have from time to time drawn between the two hospitals. In my discussion of the units, as in my discussions of doctors, nurses, patients, and families, I have been as much interested in the range of styles as in discovering a single, invariant style. In this respect, I was fortunate to have Outerboro and Countryside as my two cases. My good fortune was, in part, the result of design. My decision to study one unit in New York and another in Massachusetts was part of an altogether self-conscious effort to see the effects of different legal contexts. But my good fortune was, even more, the result of accident. The greater willingness of Outerboro physicians to extend their efforts at the end of life and the greater emphasis of Countryside physicians on the allocation of scarce resources was not a variation I had anticipated when I began my research. Yet, whether from design or accident, the differences between the two units establish a range of possibilities. Moreover, precisely because the two units differ in critical respects, it is all the more convincing that those practices they do share are general to medicine as a whole.

General Index

247

Index of Doctors, Nurses, Patients, and Families of Patients